Carnage in America

Covid-19, Racial Injustice, and the Demise of Donald Trump

Steven Weiss, M.D.

CONTENTS

INTRODUCTION

I'm a doctor. Sixty-two years old. Three grown children.

After medical school graduation and an internship in Kentucky, I flew to Honolulu (tough duty, I know) for my residency training. The city has a sizable gay population, and I learned how to care for patients with AIDS.

In 1988, when I moved back to my home town of Eau Claire, Wis., word got out that I had an interest in AIDS. My patients, all men, either were gay or had hemophilia. They suffered from unusual infections in their brains, eyes, or lungs. Typically, the infections were treatable, but the virus wasn't; drug cocktails that changed AIDS from a death sentence to a chronic disease didn't arrive until the mid-90s. The young men, in that pre-drug era, wasted away mentally and physically. Often abandoned by their families, they died alone.

Clinically devastating and unique biologically, AIDS also became political. Even as HIV was killing them, gay men fought for effective treatment.

A Republican president wasn't listening. He refused to give the virus due respect. Not until autumn of 1985 did Ronald Reagan publicly discuss AIDS. Perhaps he was heeding religious conservatives who called AIDS a gay curse, God's just and deserved punishment.

I'm haunted by plagues.

So when word came of a contagion in China, in a city named Wuhan, my brain went on high alert. Soon after, I sat in a Maui conference room attending an internal medicine update, where the first doctor's topic was new developments in infectious disease.

"I had to tweak my talk a bit," he said. "Figured I should share something regarding this virus we've all been hearing about."

There were ripples of laughter across the room.

By mid-February, it was clear to me that virus-wrought mayhem would only get worse. I read all things COVID, to which my wife can attest. On March 22, sensing that 2020 would be momentous, I started a daily diary. Ten days later, my son Erik, a tech-savvy millennial, turned my chronicle into the blog that became this book.

Heroism amidst tragedy. Missed opportunities and breathtaking incompetence. Heartache leavened with moments of joy.

I'll be your tour guide, but the journey is ours. Americans each of us, we've endured it together.

NOW WE WAIT

March 22, 2020

In early January, we heard about an outbreak of a novel coronavirus in Wuhan, China, a city of 11 million. Over the ensuing weeks, as the epidemic worsened and I watched my Chinese counterparts struggle against a contagious and sometimes lethal disease, I was humbled by their dedication and heroism. More than 3,300 Chinese health care workers were infected with the virus and at least 18 have died.

In the last two weeks, the virus has outpaced all efforts to contain it. It took three months for the world to record 100,000 cases, 12 days for the next 100,000, just three more to breach the 300,000 mark.

I practice internal medicine at Mayo-Eau Claire. Forty-eight hours ago, in an all-staff email, our leadership told us, "This is not business as usual. We are in the midst of an event without precedent." Last night, we were told, "We are in an unprecedented time. We are making decisions that we would have never imagined." Visitors are now banned from the clinic and hospital. Exceptions include one visitor for end of life care, the birth of a child, or pediatric patients. Starting tomorrow, all staff must take their temperature twice a day. Anyone with a fever exceeding 100.3 degrees, or other possible coronavirus symptoms, cannot work. For at least the next eight weeks, vacations are prohibited.

To protect patients and staff, only essential surgeries, procedures, and outpatient visits will proceed as scheduled. We'll be calling patients on the phone or, when possible, doing videoconferences. Only patients with urgent problems, who must be seen face-to-face to prevent hospitalization, will be seen per routine. We've been instructed to stay six feet away from everyone, in the clinic and out, including co-workers, and to avoid all social gatherings.

For 27 years, I was a traditional internist, seeing patients in the clinic and making rounds on them in the hospital. Four and a half years ago, our internal medicine department decided to move to the clinic alone. Anticipating a surge of inpatients, our hospitalist colleagues have asked for help, should it be necessary. Because I'd feel more useful, I've added my name to the list.

Like me, millions of Americans want to chip in. A friend has reached out to shop and run errands for elders, who risk worse consequences from the virus. My wife will be delivering meals on wheels.

To prevent health care workers from being infected, N95 masks work best. But there aren't enough, so we've been told to use regular surgical masks until, according to the CDC, the supply chain for producing them can be reestablished.

Meanwhile, POTUS dithers and distracts and blames everyone else. But according to a poll done two days ago, 55 percent of Americans approve of his handling of the pandemic. In a crisis, leaders accrue power. Remember the Patriot Act, in the wake of 9-11, which passed the Senate with just one dissenting vote?

In a recent press conference, when POTUS hyped hydroxychloroquine and azithromycin as a COVID treatment, Dr. Anthony Fauci stared down at his shoes. Later, after Dr. Fauci tried to tamp down expectations, POTUS got the last word. "I don't know," he said. "I'm a smart guy, and I've got a good feeling about this. We'll see."

Dr. Fauci has had to walk a fine line between truth-telling and deference to POTUS's ego. Today, on CBS *Face the Nation*, he praised POTUS's decision to limit travel from China and Europe, though most epidemiologists don't believe such restrictions hinder a pandemic's spread; certainly for COVID, it didn't work. But Fauci, who *really* is a smart guy, knows he needs to flatter POTUS to get his ear, so perhaps he can be nudged toward taking steps to mitigate the virus's toll.

Blue states on the coasts, urban areas in particular, especially New York City, have been hardest hit. In general—thus far—red states have been relatively spared. Since red states are more rural, social-distanced geographically, this isn't unexpected, nor is it strange that the 25 states that have yet to ban indoor dining in restaurants are exclusively red. But POTUS and his friends at Fox and on right-wing radio have downplayed COVID for weeks, leading Republicans to take the virus less seriously than Democrats. When all is said and done, will red states endure more suffering than blue states?

I've become a pariah. Because I work in health care, two of my friends want to stay away from me, avoiding even walking outside. I'm not mad. Better to be too scared of the virus than not frightened enough. I bought groceries last night, and the store I went to wasn't facilitating social distancing, so I emailed a colleague at the health department.

In America this winter, we've had 45 million flu cases contributing to 40,000 deaths. COVID is three times more contagious and 10 times more lethal. Four days ago, standing in front of a local Kwik Trip, two seventy-something men smoked and talked and disparaged the "liberals" bent on destroying the economy. Afterwards, one got in his truck, rolled down the window, and spat a big glob of phlegm on the sidewalk in front of the entrance.

In the wake of Hurricane Katrina, I worked in a Red Cross shelter set up for evacuees south of Baton Rouge. When Hurricane Rita came through, I was asked to coordinate medical care for 500 Lake Charles-area residents holed up in a school. The path of the hurricane had been broadcast for days, but I was surprised at how many people had not brought with them essential medicines for serious conditions such as seizures or heart problems.

It feels like that now, the calm before the storm. The path of a hurricane, its relentless approach, even when shown by satellite images, some people deny. Doctors and nurses and concerned citizens in western Wisconsin feel the rising winds of the oncoming storm. But not everyone shares our sensibility.

We've tried to prepare. Now we wait.

TO OUR PATIENTS: STAY AWAY!

March 23

There was an eerie scene this morning when I walked into work. Our waiting room, which I share with 12 providers, was empty, each at-least-six-feet-from-another chair unoccupied. We're trying to keep patients out of the clinic, for their safety and ours.

It's working. This morning I saw only two patients in the clinic. Other interactions were handled over the phone.

I'm less on edge at work, where having a purpose translates into less free-floating anxiety. Later this week, I'll be rounding with a hospitalist, to get up to speed on the inpatient electronic health record (EHR).

My colleague at the health department tells me they're distributing a flyer jointly with the Chamber of Commerce urging grocery stores to stress social distancing. Looking ahead, grocery and convenience stores are potential sites for the virus to spread. This morning, I called the manager of my grocery store to reinforce the message.

Tomorrow, my 89-year-old parents will drive back to Wisconsin from Florida. Their ages put their risk of death from COVID at 20 percent. I've asked them to keep their distance from people in gas stations, walk in and out of bathrooms quickly—as fast as near nonagenarians can—and eat in their motel rooms. When they get home, my wife or I will buy their groceries.

Meanwhile, POTUS, in a midnight tweet storm, said, "WE CANNOT LET THE CURE"—the White House advisory to keep group sizes at ten or less and maintain social distancing (even as this latter recommendation is regularly flouted by the COVID task force) set to expire a week from today—"BE WORSE THAN THE PROBLEM ITSELF. AT THE END OF THE 15 DAY PERIOD WE WILL MAKE A DECISION AS TO WHICH WAY WE WANT TO GO!" And Dr. POTUS continues to push an unproven drug to treat COVID at a time when tighter restrictions are essential to prevent its spread.

POTUS keeps his eye on the numbers, in particular his approval rating. The majority of Americans commend his pandemic work, so he thinks, "Go, me!"

Dr. Fauci's job keeps getting tougher. POTUS blames China for not telling the world about COVID last autumn, when no one knew what was going on. (The truth is that, in late December, the Chinese were secretive, but Chinese researchers published the virus's RNA sequence January 9.) When confronted with Trump's disinformation, Fauci said, "I can't jump in front of the microphone and push him down." When asked if he was criticized for putting his hands over his face in reaction to one of POTUS's whoppers, the doctor replied, "No comment."

3M sent 500,000 N95 masks to New York, where there's a desperate need. Despite intense pressure to invoke the Defense Production Act to protect health care workers from COVID—eight percent of Italy's 64,000 cases are health care workers—POTUS refuses; big business has lobbied against the act, saying it would impose red tape on companies when they need flexibility to navigate closed borders and shuttered factories.

The significance of Republican votes to acquit POTUS of impeachment charges has never been more apparent. Can Dr. Fauci appeal to the 25th Amendment?

To deal with the tragedy in Wuhan, the Chinese sent more than 40,000 health care workers to the city and built two hospitals in a matter of days. They'd learned their lesson from the initial outbreak; everyone wore N95 masks, two gowns, eye protection, gloves, and shoe covers. After their shifts in the hospital, this personal protective equipment (PPE) was doffed in designated areas. None of these doctors and nurses was infected with COVID. Can Americans be this disciplined? Will the nation mobilize to equip health care workers with adequate PPE?

I'm the board president at our local free clinic, where I work with an excellent team. Last week, I triaged patients at the door, to ensure no one with COVID symptoms entered the clinic. (Had there been any, they would have been directed to Eau Claire's drive-through test site, or the ER, depending on how sick they were.) Tomorrow, I'll do the same, turning away patients whose problems aren't serious. Volunteers are canceling. It's unclear how long, and under what circumstances, we can stay open, though we'll continue to provide medicines to our 600 established patients, offering curbside pickup or mailing them out.

For lunch, I had a cup of soup and an apple in an empty doctor's lounge, usually a hub of activity. I washed my hands before I ate. Most sinks have automatic faucets, but not in the lounge. My elbow, with difficulty, shut the water off.

Concern about contact with contaminated surfaces can get out of control. Who's touched that door handle? Up and down stairs, I'm walking railing-less.

Geoff Dyer ran with this in a recent *New Yorker* article. He and his tennis partner have quit their post-match handshake. But what to do about the tennis balls that both of them touch?

Said Dyer, "A friend who teaches Faulkner saw exactly what I was up to as I Englishly ushered him ahead ("Please, after you, Brian"), but he stepped up and reached for the bug-smeared door anyway. Naturally, he was up to something, too, and had taken measures to insure that *As I lay Dying* remained a literary rather than literal experience. He was holding the door for me because he was also, in drug argot, holding. Hand sanitizer, that is."

The head of the St. Louis Fed says that GDP may be cut in half and unemployment may reach 30 percent.

Four patients in the county have tested positive for COVID, and seven more are under investigation in our hospital. Though it's estimated that 11 times more people are infected than have tested positive, there's still hope that, at least in Eau Claire, the curve of infections over time will be more or less flat. If everyone other than essential workers sheltered in place for two weeks, and if essential workers paid meticulous attention to infection control, the virus would disappear.

If only we could do it.

DR. POTUS VS. PUBLIC HEALTH

March 24

Dr. Fauci was absent for the press briefing yesterday. Perhaps this was because POTUS pivoted to the economy—"Our country wasn't built to be shut down. America will, again, and soon, be open for business"—or maybe because Fauci had dared to criticize POTUS, who says that if it was up to doctors, they'd shut down the world.

Dr. POTUS calls hydroxychloroquine a "game changer" and "a gift from God," based on a small and inconclusive French study of 26 patients. Of six patients "lost to follow up," one died and three went to critical care centers different from the enrolling hospital, but Dr. Oz is impressed.

In Africa and Haiti, hydroxychloroquine is used to prevent and treat malaria. In the U.S., patients with lupus and rheumatoid arthritis (RA) take it. Unscrupulous doctors are writing prescriptions for themselves and their families, shrinking a finite supply, so lupus and RA patients can't fill their prescriptions.

Oh, Dr. POTUS.

In a matter of days, social distancing has morphed into social anxiety, not so much fear of the other but of the other coming too close. Ten days ago, as my wife and I walked beside the Chippewa, on the bike trail in downtown

Eau Claire, a young man rode toward us, extended his arms—look mom, no hands!—and said, "Welcome to the apocalypse!" Strangers greeted each other with smiles and hellos. Yesterday, curt nods had replaced the grins, as if a more welcoming expression might encourage stopping and talking. The dour expressions of the bikers and walkers matched the gray skies.

In Germany, a 33-year-old man licked the railings and a ticket machine in the subway, hoping to infect others with COVID. In England, three teenagers coughed in the faces of an elderly couple. In Spain, frail residents of care homes were abandoned and left to die; the staff had no access to PPE. In Texas, the Lieutenant Governor suggested that exposing older people to COVID, even if they died as a result, might be justified by the benefits to the economy.

Giuseppe Berardelli, a 72-year-old Italian priest, gave a ventilator purchased for him by his parishioners to a younger man he'd never met before succumbing to the virus. In Italy, COVID has killed 50 priests.

Adam Gopnik, writing yesterday in *The New Yorker*, said that "cities are always organisms of a kind, like coral reefs, where a lot of people come together to barter spices and exchange ideas and find mates, and endure the recurrent damage of infectious disease. Emptiness and absence," he writes, "contradict the very concept of the city."

Closer to home, there's a glimmer of hope. In Wisconsin, case increases the last two days total less than 80, compared to 100 in the previous 24 hours. In Eau Claire County, cases remained at four these last 48 hours. Thus far, all of the patients in our Eau Claire hospital under investigation for COVID have tested negative. We're preparing for a COVID surge but hope it won't materialize, a hope that seems more realistic than just a day ago. Time will tell.

Stanford's John Ioannidis, a prominent physician-epidemiologist, suggests that the death rate, expressed as fatalities/total cases, may be lower than is commonly thought, because the true denominator is much higher than the number of positive tests; it's been estimated that U.S. cases, currently approaching 50,000, are actually ten times higher. Ioannidis notes that Iceland has extensively tested its citizens—there are less than 400,000—and found a prevalence of the virus of one percent, half of whom have no symptoms. South Korea has tested its population extensively, 30 times more per capita than the U.S., and their data suggest that 99 percent of patients have mild or no symptoms. Knowing the true prevalence of infection in assorted parts of the country would let public health specialists better protect the nation's well-being, targeting preventive measures to regional outbreaks while mitigating adverse economic effects. At least that's the hope.

But a tradeoff between public health and unemployment is a luxury we can't currently afford. New York City has seen 5,500 new cases in the last 24 hours and more than 100 additional deaths. Each three days, cases double in the city. Harvard epidemiologist Mark Lipsitch says restricting social interactions today won't decrease ICU hospitalizations for three weeks, the time from inhaling someone's expectorated virus-laden droplets until you yourself become critically ill.

POTUS wants the country open again by Easter Sunday, a symbolism he hopes won't be lost on his flock. "We're near the end of our historic battle against the invisible enemy," he says. "Packed churches on Easter Sunday would be a beautiful thing."

The country ought to be closing instead. When the Chinese realized there was an epidemic, they locked down Hubei, the province of 60 million surrounding Wuhan. Although the Vice President has encouraged recent travelers through NYC to self-quarantine for two weeks, no one is considering cordoning off the metropolis; according to Expedia, 80 flights are scheduled from LaGuardia to Minneapolis on Easter Sunday, starting at $63 roundtrip. Like last week's spring breakers cavorting on Florida's beaches, the virus will accompany these travelers home.

As I write, that's what they're doing. Many are returning to red states where bars and restaurants remain open, where they'll unwittingly infect other patrons with a virus that has yet to, and may not ever, make them sick.

WHAT DO GOD'S PEOPLE HAVE TO SAY?

March 25

In the coming weeks, New York City is poised to become the pandemic's epicenter, the worst hit region in the world. The outbreak there has been traced to a lawyer in New Rochelle who unknowingly spread the virus through contacts at his synagogue.

In South Korea, thousands of cases were traced to a 61-year-old super spreader who was a member of Shincheonji, a Christian sect with more than a quarter million members.

In the midst of a pandemic, where is God?

In 2001, I attended a church on the south side of Eau Claire. On the evening of 9/11, the pastor held an impromptu and well-attended service. In a crisis, people congregate for mutual support. They amassed in the Middle Ages, during pestilences past, magnifying the risk of contagion. Then and now, believers assemble in churches and mosques and synagogues. It would be nice, as POTUS says, to have churches on Easter Sunday filled to the brim.

But wishing won't make it so. Unfortunately, some pastors and many of their parishioners take POTUS at his word. As a consequence, more people will die.

In a pandemic, where are God's emissaries? What are they saying and doing? We've heard about Italy's priests. On the other hand, there's Jerry Falwell, Jr., a POTUS stalwart, who on *Fox and Friends* recently said, "You remember the North Korean leader promised a Christmas present for America? Could it be they got together with China and this is that present? I don't know. But it really is something strange going on here." None of the hosts challenged this baseless theory.

Falwell has compared COVID to the flu, which doesn't rampage through a nursing home, killing 35 of its 120 residents, as happened in Kirkland, Wash. He's accused the media of stoking fear. He was late to shut down Liberty University earlier this month; yesterday, disregarding the entreaties of public health authorities, he welcomed 1,700 Liberty students back to campus, where classes will also be offered online. Not science but God— rather, Falwell's conception of a deity—is his authority.

On March 13, I had dinner with the local pastor mentioned above, who despite my atrophied faith is still a close friend. I chose an uncrowded restaurant for the last restaurant meal I expect to eat in months, and we sat at a secluded booth in the back. Earlier in the day, he'd emailed wondering if the societal response to COVID was under-reaction, over-reaction, or just right. I replied that, at long last, we were coming to grips with the problem's magnitude. His church, Eau Claire's largest, has begun a six-million-dollar capital campaign. Commitment Sunday was in two days.

He cancelled the services.

Yesterday, I suffered through a three-hour virtual training in order to use the inpatient EHR. The next two days, to further familiarize myself with the software, I'll be rounding with a hospitalist. Today, my day off, I stopped by my office for my N95 in case it's needed tomorrow. Wisconsin COVID cases increased today by 129 to 585 total, the state's largest single-day rise, but cases in Eau Claire inched up from only four to five, with no COVID-positive inpatients in any of our five northwest Wisconsin hospitals.

In Eau Claire, we're still concerned about a patient surge. Our CEO co-wrote a piece in the NY Times arguing against opening schools and businesses. The economy won't recover, he and six other health care leaders agree, until the pandemic ends. The leaders have modeled expectations for a surge in critically ill patients that suggests if a hospital has 25 COVID-positive patients, with two in the ICU and one of these on a ventilator, 800 patients might need a ventilator one month later.

Because of rigorous infection control efforts, combined with fine work by local public health specialists and proactive steps by Governor Tony Evers, together with a low burden of infection in northwest Wisconsin—Eau Claire, population ~ 70,000, is the largest city—our region might not see a surge. With luck and/or the grace of God, our curve might be somewhat flat. But we don't know.

What *is* clear is that New York City is experiencing a tragedy. Elmhurst Hospital in the Bronx reported 13 COVID deaths in the past 24 hours. Dr. Ashley Bray, a 27-year-old internal medicine resident, described doing CPR on a woman in her eighties, a man in his sixties, and a 38-year-old man who reminded her of her fiancé. All had COVID, each patient died. Twenty-eight hundred COVID patients are currently hospitalized across the city. Forty-eight hours from now, the city's 1,800 ICU beds are projected to be full. Governor Andrew Cuomo has put out a plea for retired RNs to return to work. More doctors will be needed, too.

RED OR BLUE STATE, COVID DOESN'T DISCRIMINATE

March 26

We have the first COVID case in our hospital. He's a frail man in his 70s from a small, rural town. He lives alone and is helped by a caregiver. Neither he nor his attendant had recently traveled outside of the area. There was a gathering at his home 12 days earlier, where someone, it's presumed, infected him. In the last week, before coming to our hospital, he was seen by two other clinics. How many health care workers and patients might have been exposed? I talked with the attending physician and encouraged him to wear an N95 mask, even though our institutional guideline states a surgical mask, together with a face shield and gown and gloves, protects sufficiently. We need to conserve N95s, we're told; there's a nationwide shortage.

There's a new feel to the hospital. Every doctor and nurse wears a mask, doors are opened with elbows, computer mice and keyboards wiped clean.

Louisiana has the fastest growing COVID surge in the world. Their first case was diagnosed March 9, but epidemiologists believe the outbreak started in New Orleans over Mardi Gras, which concluded on Feb. 25. The state has over 2,300 cases, and at least 83 patients have died. Mardi Gras has been compared to the infamous "Liberty Loan" parade in Philadelphia, in 1918, when, at the height of the influenza pandemic, 200,000 people jammed the streets. Six weeks later, the flu had killed 12,000 Philadelphians.

Within days of Louisiana's first case, Gov. John Bel Edwards, a Democrat, shut schools and banned large gatherings, including the huge St. Patrick's Day parade. One week after the first case, he closed all bars and restaurants—a sharp contrast with his neighboring states. Republican Mississippi Gov. Tate Reaves said he rejects "dictatorship models like China." His "executive order" to ostensibly address the COVID crisis exempts most businesses, public and private, deeming all of them "essential." To the east, Governor Kay Ivey, another Republican, echoes POTUS. "The safety and well-being of Alabamians is paramount," she says. "However, I agree with President Trump who thinks that a healthy and vital economy is just as essential to our quality of life." At present, 21 states are under shelter-in-place orders. Fifteen are blue, six are red. Ohio Governor Mike DeWine and Maryland Governor Larry Hogan have emerged as Republican leaders in the fight against COVID.

In 2014, during an Ebola outbreak in Sierra Leone, researchers discovered an interesting phenomenon. More Ebola cases were reported in parts of the country where people had greater trust in the government and the health care system than in those with less trust. Why? People believed the government and the health care system would take care of them.

And they did. In regions with greater trust, though more cases were diagnosed, there were fewer deaths.

Will something similar occur with COVID? In Mississippi, if people trust Governor Reaves and POTUS more than doctors and epidemiologists? In Louisiana, if they favor the vicissitudes of POTUS instead of science-based rules?

One such Louisianan is Pastor Tony Spell of Life Tabernacle Church in Baton Rouge, who defied a state mandate Sunday by hosting 1100 parishioners. "It's not a concern," Spell says. "The virus, we believe, is politically motivated. We hold our religious rights dear and we are going to assemble no matter what someone says."

In the United States, state government plays the primary role in public health emergencies, and the lack of a strong, centrally coordinated public health authority, independent of POTUS, has never glared more.

Hospitals are discussing not resuscitating patients with COVID even if they or their families want CPR; CPR generates aerosols, which put resuscitation teams at risk. Dr. Lewis Kaplan, president of the Society of Critical Care Medicine, says "we are on a crisis footing. What you take as first-come, first-served, no-holds-barred, everything-that-is-available-should-be-applied medicine is not where we are."

University of Wisconsin bioethicist R. Alta Charo adds that the idea of withholding treatments, though unsettling—especially in wealthy countries like the United States—is practical. "It doesn't help anybody if our doctors and nurses are felled by this virus and not able to care for us," she says. "The code process is one that puts them at enhanced risk." In Spain, more than 10,000 of 80,000 COVID cases have occurred in health care workers.

Contagion in hospitals can go both ways. In mid-19th century Budapest, women died of sepsis at horrific rates after giving birth; obstetricians and the men doing autopsies—one and the same—refused to wash their hands, despite the repeated urgings of Ignaz Semmelweis, after whom Hungary's most prominent medical school is named. Our doctors and nurses, if meticulous infection control procedures aren't followed, also may make patients sick.

FROM A FOUNDATION OF FEAR, BARRICADES ARISE

March 27

The last two days, I've taken my temperature while driving to work. There's no beep when it's done, as advertised; at red lights I steal glances at the thermometer. Temperatures can be taken, per the package insert, in mouth, rectum, or armpit. I told our clinic nurses I'm rotating sites. Then I asked Nancy, the nurse I've worked with for 32 years, "How many times have you wanted to tell me to eat shit?"

We have our second COVID case in the hospital. It's palpable, a heightened sense of anxiety, more pronounced in the younger docs. Before we head out on rounds, Kosta Talitsky, M.D., swabs his computer mouse and keyboard meticulously with an alcohol wipe. Dr. Talitsky, from Moscow, Russia, also has a Ph.D. in cardiovascular cell biology. He's tall, medium build, in his late thirties, with thinning black hair—and computer skills that dwarf mine. He wears blue scrubs over a white t-shirt, black-rimmed glasses, and Asics on his feet. I'm shadowing him in the hospital to learn the inpatient EHR in case I'm needed in the event of a surge.

Dr. Talitsky got a call to the emergency room to admit a patient with symptoms suspicious for COVID, and we geared up outside room 10: gown, blue nitrile gloves, face shields affixed to masks. Dr. Talitsky kindly informed me my shield/mask was upside down. That this style wouldn't keep respiratory droplets out of my eyes he let me decipher myself.

The patient was a Hmong woman in her sixties who receives peritoneal dialysis because of kidney failure. She lives with her son, who works at 3M and was sent home because of exposure to a co-worker diagnosed with COVID. Dr. Talitsky ordered a nasal swab on our patient for the virus.

We went up to the floor, where our next patient was an overweight white woman taking a blood thinner who'd been admitted for a large intra-abdominal bleed. She'd had influenza two and a half weeks earlier. Yesterday afternoon, her cough returned.

She's bringing up sputum, a favorable sign. COVID damages the lining of the alveoli, the air sacs in the lung, more than summoning white cells to *within* the alveoli, so the cough is dry and no sputum is produced. She doesn't have a fever and isn't short of breath. It's unlikely the patient has COVID, but she, too, will be tested. The more COVID you see, the more COVID you think you do.

In the last week, China has had more cases of the virus from international travelers than have been diagnosed domestically. In fact, few cases of in-country transmission have occurred. Yesterday, the government limited all airlines to one flight into China each week.

It's ironic. Two months ago, the Chinese complained bitterly about POTUS's decision to restrict flights from China to the United States, in part because this ran counter to WHO's guidance. Mayo has banned new hires from outside of the enterprise. Whether or not such restrictions are wise isn't known. But one thing is certain. In this pandemic, nations and institutions are building barricades and hunkering down.

As has POTUS's America, erecting virtual walls instead of the literal one on which he campaigned. Come November, it might work. Eighty-six percent of Republicans approve of his handling of the pandemic, and independents seem to be moving his way—the rally effect.

Then again, all things COVID move fast. Ravages to the economy, swings of the market, the virus itself. Wouldn't political effects be similar, at least among the 20 percent of Americans who about POTUS might yet be persuadable?

As countries and companies close themselves off, POTUS wants America to open up. Backing away from making the U.S. unsafer still on Easter, POTUS now says he'll divide the nation into regions of risk: "low," "medium," and "high." "I think we can start by opening up…the farm belt, certain parts of the Midwest, other places," he said.

The man who knew more about ISIS than the generals knows more about COVID than the epidemiologists. The director of the Harvard Global Health Initiative, Dr. Ashish Jha, says, "We are in for a bumpy ride for the next 12 to 18 months. If we are aggressive now about stopping things, shutting down, building up a test regime, we can then open up again…and most places can go back to work. But only when we are ready," he added. "And we are nowhere near ready now."

The emperor without any clothes? More like King Lear, a madman leading the blind.

More ironies. Boris Johnson, POTUS's COVID-threat-minimizing-comrade across the pond, is sick with the virus.

In her book *On Immunity*, Eula Bliss describes an innate wariness of outside groups—immigrants, minorities, people with disabilities—a hardwired disease prevention strategy that alerts us to unfamiliar behavior or physical difference, harmless though they typically are, a rationale for raising the proverbial walls. Evolutionary psychologists explain that this "behavioral immune system" peaks when people are most vulnerable. In the first trimester of pregnancy, for example, women exhibit increased xenophobia. Syphilis was the French pox to the English, *morbus Germanicus* to Parisians, the Naples sickness to Florentines, while the Japanese called it the Chinese disease.

In a study done at the height of the 2009 H1N1 influenza pandemic, people in vaccinated and unvaccinated groups were asked to read an article that amplified the pandemic's threats. Later, they completed a survey assessing their attitudes toward immigrants. The vaccinated subjects were less prejudiced. The researchers delved deeper, defining vaccination as either "the seasonal flu vaccine involves injecting people with the seasonal flu virus" or "the seasonal flu vaccine protects people from the seasonal flu." The former phrasing increased xenophobia, while the latter language didn't.

Wouldn't it be nice to vaccinate people against biases in addition to viruses? Let POTUS be inoculated first.

THINKING, AND
PRECEDENT

March 28

In metro areas across the country, the pandemic is accelerating. Philadelphia and Milwaukee have hundreds of cases, Dallas and Houston, too. Each city sits on the front end of a sharply increasing curve. In Detroit, Los Angeles, and Chicago, cases exceed 1,000, stressing nurses and doctors and hospitals. Two hundred thirteen U.S. cities complain of not having enough PPE and/or ventilators. Finally, after weeks of unrelenting pressure, POTUS ordered GM to start making masks and ventilators. It will be two weeks before they start production. Meanwhile, health care workers will be infected, and some will die.

Instead of leadership, POTUS rebukes and ridicules. Last night, he tweeted, "I love Michigan, one of the reasons we are doing such a great job for them during this horrible Pandemic. Yet your Governor, Gretchen "Half'" Whitmer is way over her head, she doesn't have a clue. Likes blaming everyone for her own ineptitude." If POTUS had looked in the mirror while tweeting, truer words he'd never said. He's told Vice President Pence to not return governors' calls if they don't show him due appreciation.

Yesterday, Mayo revealed our surge plan. If the surge happens, the ICU will be dedicated to COVID patients, and the post-anesthesia care unit and cath lab will house patients without COVID who are critically ill. Fourth floor south will care for patients under investigation (PUI) for COVID and any who've tested positive. When COVID numbers increase, they'll be housed on 4N, with PUIs moved to 4S. When these cohorts are fully separate, to conserve scarce PPE, the entirety of 4S will become a negative pressure unit.

Flatten the curve. Even people with an aversion to math and an abhorrence of graphs get the goal. But how to do it? Are there lessons to be gleaned from history?

Only a few centenarians have any memory of the 1918 influenza pandemic. The first known U.S. case occurred in March, 1918, at a Kansas military base. From there, the epidemic spread quickly across the country. Philadelphia saw its first case Sept. 17. The next day, city officials launched a campaign against public coughing, sneezing, or spitting.

Yet 10 days later, they hosted a parade attended by 200,000 people. Flu cases climbed. By Oct. 3, when the city finally shut down churches, schools, and theaters, more than 20,000 people had taken sick. Six weeks after the parade, the flu had killed 12,000 Philadelphians.

Of 43 American cities studied, 24 weeks into their local epidemics, Philadelphia's mortality rate was highest. In contrast, New York City began quarantine measures 11 days *before* a spike in deaths and had the lowest mortality rate on the East Coast.

Not only is it important when in the curve social distancing regulations were implemented, but their duration also mattered. St. Louis had strong social distancing regulations and a low total death rate, but they suffered a sharp increase, a second peak higher than the first, when the restrictions were prematurely relaxed.

Forty-two of 43 cities endured a second peak. Fall River, Mass., for unknown reasons, was the sole exception. In general, the height of the second peak was inversely proportional to the duration of social distancing.

The info above was taken from today's *National Geographic*. Barack Obama, or Hillary Clinton, would have already read the article and absorbed its lessons. But it'll fly beneath POTUS's radar, nor will he have patience for anyone hazarding to inform him of the article.

For many working class Americans, POTUS is their middle finger, disdaining the advice of elites. Anti-intellectualism in American life has a long history, as described by Richard Hofstadter in his 1963 Pulitzer Prize-winning book. As Frederick Jackson Turner noted, more than anything in U.S. history, the conquest of the western frontier forged our character. We're a nation of doers, starting with the immigrants who boarded ships bound for America, accompanied only by their hopes and dreams, and including Africans taken here forcibly, who worked hardest and suffered most. A real estate developer's instincts—"I'm a smart guy, and I've got a good feeling about this drug, a better feeling than Dr. Fauci"—or the science-based perspective of an epidemiologist? No contest, for POTUS's core.

Harvard professor and Pulitzer Prize-winning author Louis Menand further explains POTUS's appeal. When we buy a stereo, for instance, few of us know the costs and performance of the vast array of possible components. Instead, we rely on a friend's take and a salesperson's spiel. Most of us, according to Menand's review of the relevant literature, take a similar shortcut, or heuristic, when deciding for whom we should vote. We listen to commentators in our media silos, perhaps an informed and/or charismatic friend or family member, and add our hunches to make up our minds. Remember Michael Dukakis in a helmet, riding around in a tank? George H.W. Bush not knowing grocery store scanners were a thing? Our emotional reactions helped us decide for whom to vote.

The majority of our thinking, loosely defined, according to Nobel Prize-winning psychologist Daniel Kahneman, author of the best-selling *Thinking, Fast and Slow*, is instinctual. When we drive home from work, for example, seldom are we consciously aware of the other cars on the road. It's similar in medicine. The longer your career, the more accurate are the diagnoses you formulate after the first few sentences of a patient's complaint. The challenge is to push past these initial impressions, consider other possibilities, and perform the hard work of thinking slowly.

We need a leader who can do that, and do it well. Instead, we have POTUS. The latest? As would be expected, people are fleeing COVID hotbeds such as New York and New Orleans, refugees from the former sometimes decamping for Florida, whose governor has ordered them quarantined for 14 days. POTUS is said to be mulling "an enforceable quarantine" of New York, New Jersey, and parts of Connecticut.

Why stop there? 19 days ago, Italy locked down. Their curve is eight days ahead of ours. To have a chance at emerging from the pandemic less scathed than Italy, we should have locked down two weeks ago.

I'm worried about patients without COVID who will fall through the cracks. Yesterday afternoon, I drove to a rural nursing home to see a patient I've taken care of for decades, a lady in her 90s bedridden by MS. She'd been vomiting and had an infected ulcer on her leg. Because of COVID, my patient is confined to a nursing home.

Today, Saturday, I made a house call on a patient and friend, a man who went home two and a half weeks ago after months of institutional care. He has diabetes, and a foot to which, in mid-October, blood clots had traveled, leaving three toes—one has been amputated—with gangrene.

Later, I stopped to see a high school buddy who'd contacted me earlier complaining of a bulge in his groin. Unless the hernia becomes life-threatening, he'll have to live with it. Any elective surgery, no matter how elective is defined, has been put on hold. Most of our surgeons are working from home to guard against exposure to the virus. Starting next week, all but four of our fourteen internists, for the same reason, will do the same.

FOX AND FRIENDS

March 29

My cousin and I began fishing together on family vacations five decades ago. After graduation from college at UW-Superior—he started on the football team each of his four years and as a senior was named captain—he flew F4 fighters in the Air Force for seven years. After his military service, he flew for the DNR before joining American Airlines, where he retired as a captain. He's active in his church and in Wisconsin's Conservation Congress. When our beloved grandmother died at 103, he delivered a heartfelt eulogy, struggling with his emotions, while I was too choked up to speak.

Our politics are polar opposites. Most of my friends and colleagues think like me, so on occasion I reach out to him for perspective I don't often hear. On March 20, I texted him:

"Trying to gauge how my conservative cousin sees the pandemic. How big a deal is it, on a 1-10 scale? Are we doing too much to stop it, not enough, or taking just the right steps? How's Trump doing?"

He replied, "I think the so-called pandemic has become a big deal. Most of the media has called it that. I guess by now it is. Trump has done all that he can do to deal with this, starting with his early decision—much criticized, by the way—to stop travel from China to the USA back in early January (the date was January 31, when most major airlines had already suspended flights to and from China; Italy enacted a similar ban earlier the same day) after China finally let the world know what was going on over there. (The Chinese published COVID's RNA sequence January 9.) As had been noted, he inherited an outdated system that was not capable of addressing the scope of what is going on now. He is fixing it and hopefully we will be better prepared to deal with future "pandemics." Trump has taken every step necessary to clear obstacles in their path in order to come up with timely solutions. Of course the media will never give him credit for anything he does. Trump's actions to "go big" are the right actions in my opinion. I'd give him and more importantly his team a "10" for their efforts."

Later that week, he sent me a link to a post from Fox News' Shannon Bream on Bible verses she found helpful during her worst and darkest times.

Last night, we resumed our dialogue.

"We're in for the toughest two months of our lives, Joe. I know you don't see it coming. God bless…"

"I see it very plainly," he responded. "We have more cases I suppose because we've tested and continue to test more people than any other country in the world. It only figures that we would have the most cases."

"We're going to have by far the highest DEATHS in the world," I said, "and much of it was preventable. Not just the human toll. The effects on the economy will be catastrophic. And you're wrong about testing. South Korea, as of two weeks ago, had tested far more people per capita than we've tested as of now."

"Preventable by who? The Democrats? Ha-ha. All they cared about was impeaching Trump when this was happening. How'd that work out.' (The Senate voted to acquit POTUS on February 6.) 'Gloom and doom from the left. That's all we have here. If it was preventable, China should shoulder that blame for suppressing their information."

I let him have the last word.

In 1996, when Roger Ailes created Fox News, he intended to create an alternate reality, which the late Fox contributor Charles Krauthammer praised him for accomplishing. As detailed in the movie *Bombshell*, Ailes was a sexual predator. So was Bill O'Reilly. Sean Hannity has bragged about his father hitting him in the face with his fist. Abused and abusive men. Bullies. POTUS emulates the politics and behavior of the men who made Fox, which was necessary for his ascent.

If not for Roger Ailes, there'd be no Fox News, and we wouldn't be saddled with POTUS.

Mimicking POTUS, right-wing media downplays the virus's threat. Former Fox business anchor Trish Regan was fired from the network two days ago after a March 9 on-air rant: "We've reached a tipping point. The chorus of hate being leveled at President Trump is nearing a crescendo as Democrats blame him and only him for a virus that originated halfway around the world. This is yet another attempt to impeach the president."

POTUS took the occasion of her termination to defend her.

Sean Hannity, on March 11: It "may be true" that the "deep state" is using COVID to manipulate markets, suppress dissent, and push mandated medicines.

Rush Limbaugh, on February 25: "The coronavirus is being weaponized as yet another element to bring down POTUS. I want to tell you the truth about the coronavirus. Yeah, I'm dead right on this. The coronavirus is the common cold."

Limbaugh again, March 11: "Why do you think this is COVID-19? This is the 19th coronavirus." (Nineteen comes from 2019, the year the virus was discovered, having likely jumped from a bat to a pangolin and from this scaly mammal to a single human in a wet market in Wuhan, China. Seven coronaviruses are known to infect humans.) "I'll tell you what's really more scary than anything is how some Americans seem to be okay with being told they can't do this, they can't do that, and they can't go there, and you've got to stay here, and we're gonna quarantine you there, and we're gonna wrap you up over there, we're gonna put you in this cocoon here, and you can't leave and you (say)—'Okay, fine with me!' No, not okay," Limbaugh says.

Anti-science diatribes on the internet are worse. At a press conference on March 20, after POTUS referred to the "deep State Department," Dr. Fauci lowered his head and covered his face. The next day, on the internet, anti-Fauci posts proliferated, in part because of an article from *The American Thinker*, a conservative blog, which published a seven-year-old email from Fauci to Hillary Clinton praising her stamina during the Benghazi hearings. The blogger claimed this was evidence Fauci was involved in a secret anti-POTUS cabal, a baseless theory subsequently shared countless times on Facebook and Twitter.

FOR PROTECTION, TO
WHOM DO WE TURN?

March 30

In early March, with COVID spreading quickly in Washington state, members of the Skagit Valley Chorale debated whether to hold their weekly rehearsal. COVID was already killing people in Seattle, an hour south, but no cases had been detected in Skagit County, where life went on per routine.

On March 10, 60 choir members rehearsed for two and a half hours, preparing to sing late in April at the Skagit County Tulip Festival, which in non-pandemic years is attended by more than 1 million people. No one was coughing, nobody sneezed. With gusto, they belted out the first song: "Sing on! Whatever comes your way, sing on! Sing on!" Later they sang a spiritual piece penned by Gospel legend Thomas A. Dorsey: "If we ever needed the Lord before, we sure do need him now."

Three days later, several choir members came down with telltale COVID symptoms: fever, cough, shortness of breath, fatigue and achiness. Some were nauseated and had diarrhea. One woman lost her sense of taste and smell. Now, less than three weeks after the rehearsal, three quarters of the choir has COVID, and two singers are dead.

The tragedy shines light on modes of viral transmission. The WHO has downplayed aerosols as being significant and instead has focused on respiratory droplets coughed or sneezed by infected patients into the air. But aerosols may turn out to be an important means through which the virus is spread.

COVID is three times more contagious than the flu, which *is* transmitted through respiratory droplets. Might something other than the relative infectivity of these two viruses' respiratory droplets account for COVID's higher risk of contagion? At least 696 members of the NYPD are COVID positive, and three have died. Sixty-one screening TSA personnel have tested positive. Countless first responders have fallen ill.

The tragedy of the Skagit Valley Chorale casts our nationwide shortage of N95 masks, which protect against infection by aerosols, in a still more heartrending light. How did a country as wealthy as ours wind up in this predicament?

Certainly, it would have helped if POTUS had authorized the Defense Production Act weeks earlier, as he was repeatedly urged to do, and compelled private enterprise to mass produce N95 masks. And it would be nice if, instead of demeaning Democratic governors, he worked in a non-partisan way to ensure every state's health care workers had PPE to keep them safe. The role of wartime commander cherished by POTUS doesn't fit. Would he send troops into battle without helmets or functional M-16s?

Before COVID, China produced half of the world's N95s. The Chinese outbreak reduced a supply that because of wildfires in California and Australia was already precarious. China has increased production 12-fold to 115 million masks/month, claiming this domestic production for itself, even the masks made in Shanghai by 3M. Other countries have followed suit, understandably. In addition, in the last half of January, China purchased most of the world's existing mask inventory.

What can be done? 3M has doubled production of N95s to 1.1 billion per year, 400 million of which will be produced domestically. POTUS finally conscripted GM, and Nelson Laboratories and Medicom Group are pitching in.

But other problems loom. There's not enough non-woven polypropylene to make masks, forcing some factories to sit idle. Further upstream, polypropylene resin may run short, as it did during the H1N1 flu pandemic in 2009. So, for the foreseeable future, doctors and nurses face the prospect of marching into battle against a deadly enemy unequipped with adequate protective gear.

But at least POTUS has bowed to a brick of reality slapped hard against his head. When Drs. Fauci and Deborah Birx showed him a model projecting 100,000 to 200,000 U.S. deaths, even if social distancing guidelines stay in place, and deaths as high as 2.2 million if they're prematurely relaxed, POTUS shook his head and said, "I guess we've got to do it."

We needn't worry about damage to his ego. "I'm a ratings hit," he tweeted. "Since reviving the daily White House briefing I and my coronavirus updates have attracted an average audience of 8.5 million on cable news, roughly the viewership of the season finale of *The Bachelor*, and numbers are continuing to rise."

Meanwhile, in Florida, Republican Gov. Ron DeSantis has stolen a page from POTUS's playbook, quarantining visitors from outside the Sunshine State while doing little to address COVID within. At 5,700, Florida has the sixth highest number of infections in the nation, with cases doubling every three days.

Yesterday this COVID-permissive environment made it easier for a Tampa preacher to lure hundreds of parishioners to his Tampa Bay church. According to its website, "The Church is an essential service. It is a place where people turn for help and for comfort in a climate of fear and uncertainty. We believe God's word to us, which says to trust Him and to not be fearful but to have faith in Him."

The pastor, Rodney Howard-Browne, adds, "The only time this church will close is when the Rapture is taking place. We're raising up revivalists, not pansies."

AN OUNCE
OF PREVENTION

March 31

Our health care system, if system is the right term for the hodgepodge of hospitals, clinics, and nursing homes that provide care, focuses on acute problems. Nowhere else in the world can you get a hip or knee replacement as quickly as in the United States, a state-of-affairs incented by insurance companies and government, which reimburse procedures more lucratively than so-called cognitive services. In the U.S., public health is a lower priority yet, receiving only 2.5 percent of the 3.6 trillion health care dollars spent each year.

South Korea takes a different approach. Though the first cases of COVID showed up in both countries on the same date, Jan. 20, South Korea has fared far better in flattening their curve. Despite testing twice as many people per capita as the United States, South Korea has less than 10,000 cases and only 162 deaths, while the U.S. has 15 times more cases and twenty times more deaths. (South Korea, population 52 million, is less than one-sixth as big as the U.S.) More importantly, in the last 24 hours, South Korea has registered only 125 new cases and four additional deaths while America has had over 20,000 new cases and 573 more deaths. South Koreans take public health seriously. According to former FDA commissioner Scott Gottlieb, "South Korea is showing COVID can be beat with smart, aggressive public health."

Having learned from a 2015 MERS outbreak that killed 38 people, South Korea was ready for the next coronavirus to emerge. One week after their first COVID case, government officials met with reps from medical companies and prodded them to come up with a test. Two weeks later, though cases remained under 100, thousands of test kits were shipping daily. Emergency measures were imposed in Daegu, population 2.5 million, where contagion spread quickly from a church. Soon, 600 testing centers had sprung up across the country. Relentless public messaging orchestrated through strong national leadership urges citizens to be tested at the onset of COVID symptoms. Thermal image cameras screen for fevers. Restaurants check temperatures before patrons are served.

South Korea developed tools for aggressive contact tracing during the MERS outbreak, allowing health workers to trace citizens' movements using security camera footage, credit card transactions, even GPS data from cellphones and cars. A law was passed to prioritize public health over individual privacy in infectious disease crises.

Now, cellphones vibrate with alerts whenever new cases are discovered in the vicinity. Smartphone apps monitor the travel of recently infected patients, minute-to-minute, and those who may have crossed paths with them are encouraged to get a test. For violation of a quarantine order, enforced though an app that anyone infected with COVID is required to download, South Koreans face a $2,500 fine.

To subdue the outbreak, the country's leaders asked citizens for their cooperation while ensuring they were well-informed. Television broadcasts, subway station announcements, and smartphone alerts remind people to keep their distance and wear a mask.

The messaging has instilled a wartime sense of national purpose. A national health care system, which includes special provisions for COVID testing and treatment that covers everyone, further incents participation. And South Korea does this by spending only eight percent of GDP on health care, compared to 18 percent in the United States, which leaves 30 million people uninsured and tens of millions more lacking adequate coverage.

South Korea has contained COVID without shutting down the economy. Its approach and ours have led to wildly disparate results, outcomes that will further diverge in the coming months. Facing a lethal enemy, South Korea has responded with humility, while the attitude of POTUS—"We are doing a job the likes of which has never been done before"—is nothing but hubris.

The last two days I've seen a total of two patients face-to-face and made phone calls to 10 patients. (I'm not busy.) The hospital census is low. We have one COVID inpatient. He's critically ill, on a ventilator in the ICU.

In New York, Gov. Cuomo has put out a plea for doctors and nurses. "I am asking health care workers across the country. If things are not urgent in your own community, please come to New York. We need relief for doctors. If you can, help us. We will return the favor in your hour of need."

Several days ago, when I added my name to New York's volunteer site, 65,000 health care workers, including 2,000 physicians, had already registered. I love New York—like the slogan—but my employer must grant me permission to go, which seems unlikely, at least now, because of uncertainty regarding an upcoming surge.

Addendum: As of October 16, according to the website Worldometer, the U. S. has surpassed 8.2 million cases and 223,000 deaths. South Korea has had a total of 25,000 cases and a total death toll of 441. On October 16, again according to Worldometer, South Korea documented 47 additional cases and two more deaths, while the U.S. recorded 71,687 new cases and 928 added deaths.

ARE YOU
A TRADITIONALIST?

April 1

POTUS says we'll be lucky to emerge from this tragedy with 100,000 deaths. If only this were an April Fool's joke. For once, though, I agree with him. We have to play the hand we've been dealt, shitty though it is, in large part because of his mismanagement. Italy has seen more suffering from COVID—105,000 cases and over 12,000 deaths—than any other country. Their curve is seven to 10 days ahead of ours. Italy shut down more than three weeks ago, something we've yet to do.

Three weeks ago, Italians gathered on their balconies and sang *andra tutto bene* (everything will be all right.) Now, the singing has stopped, replaced by lines at food banks and social unrest.

In Spain, health care workers comprise more than 14 percent of the country's 102,000 COVID cases. In Italy, the figure is 10 percent. A doctor at an NYC hospital described it as a "petri dish" wherein more than 200 workers had fallen sick. Thomas Riley, a nurse at NYC's Jacobi Medical Center who has contracted the virus, says, "I feel like we're all just being sent to slaughter."

Yesterday, 5,600 NYPD officers were out sick, 15 percent of the force. Fourteen hundred are confirmed COVID positive. The virus has killed five policemen.

At the outset of the epidemic in Wuhan, at least 3,300 doctors and nurses fell ill. When the Chinese built two hospitals in 10 days, over 40,000 health care workers were brought in to staff them. They followed rigorous infection control practices. Everyone double gowned, wore eye protection, N95s, even foot covers. After finishing their shifts, PPE was doffed in a separate area. No health care worker caught the virus.

Why, then, are doctors and nurses getting sick and dying in Spain, Italy, and the United States?

The common wisdom of the medical community is that COVID is transmitted as is the flu, by respiratory droplets spewed by patients into the air. In addition, the virus can live on certain surfaces for up to three days.

But it's not clear the virus is transmitted often, or even ever, by contact with a virus-laden object, forgetting to wash your hands, and then touching your eyes, nose, or mouth. In my view, Dr. Deborah Birx, of the White House Coronavirus Task Force, has done the public a disservice by routinely suggesting this possibility, which diverts attention from the far more likely scenario of respiratory spread. (Dr. Oz, in his P.T. Barnum way, foments panic by encouraging people to "close the borders of their houses." Tune in to Fox for his latest COVID insights.)

We know that COVID is several times more contagious than influenza, and 10 times deadlier. Why is it more transmissible?

Patients infected with the virus, in the three days before they develop symptoms, are infectious. One study suggests that nasal carriage of COVID is actually higher in this pre-symptomatic phase than when the patient first feels sick. Some people stay without symptoms but can still pass the virus on.

A recent study in the *New England Journal of Medicine* suggests that after an infected patient leaves a room, COVID can linger in the air for three hours. TSA employees have been infected by the dozens; case reports from China suggest talking to a person who's COVID positive for less than a minute can transmit infection.

In a recent article in *Science,* researchers modeled the dynamics of COVID infection in 375 Chinese cities in the weeks before Jan. 23, when the government imposed travel restrictions. They estimate that, before that date, 86 percent of patients with symptoms significant enough to seek medical care had contracted the virus from someone who was either mildly ill or had no symptoms at all, a mode of transmission termed "undocumented." The transmission rate of such infections was 55 percent the rate of "documented" infections between symptomatic individuals. Yet due to their much higher numbers at the outset of the epidemic, undocumented infections caused four-fifths of all new infections.

As I build my case, I have two more points. Research from the National Strategic Research Institute at the University of Nebraska further suggests that COVID can be transmitted through a so-called airborne mechanism, as is measles, though COVID, fortunately, is several times less communicable. Samples gathered from isolation rooms of COVID patients had high levels of viral contamination in the air, and air samples from hallways outside of the rooms were also positive. For COVID, PPE for airborne pathogens may be appropriate, the researchers said.

Forty-four of 60 choir members contracted COVID from an asymptomatic or mildly symptomatic colleague. This supports transmission by aerosol; singing generates more aerosol than simple speech.

Both the CDC and the WHO downplay aerosol as an important mechanism for COVID transmission. Both organizations say a regular surgical mask, rather than an N95, protects sufficiently. (The CDC tells nurses to use a bandanna if there aren't any masks.)

What's the difference between transmission by respiratory droplets and transmission by aerosol? When someone is infected with a respiratory virus, they emit viral particles when they talk, breathe, sneeze, or cough, particles encased in globs of mucus, saliva, and water. Bigger particles fall faster than they evaporate, so they splash down nearby in "droplet" form. Smaller globs evaporate faster than they fall, leaving dried-out virus lingering in the air and theoretically dispersible beyond the supposedly safe six-foot radius. Concerning COVID, we just don't know.

But when the WHO states that COVID "is not airborne," it's claiming the virus is spreading predominantly through close-splashing droplets that are inhaled before they hit the ground.

Taken together, what does all of this mean? From a practical perspective, should it inform policy?

The practice of medicine is a traditional enterprise. Medical students learn from interns, who learn from residents, who report to staff physicians. There's a hierarchy, which you quickly learn not to step out of. *Most* doctors do, at least.

Conservatives such as columnist George Will and Harvard political philosopher Harvey Mansfield argue that tradition, because it's traditional, is worthy of respect. (Mansfield filed an amicus brief against gay marriage when the Supreme Court considered the issue, writing that social science research purporting to show that having gay or lesbian parents fails to hurt children was produced by activists and not dispassionate scientists.) There's good reason, these men say, for societal norms to have stood the test of time. To me, the argument sounds like a tautology.

Aircraft carriers resemble large bureaucracies. Neither can turn on a dime. Both the CDC and the WHO are traditional organizations, resistant to sudden change. (Think of the slowness in the WHO's labeling COVID a pandemic on March 11 and a Public Health Emergency of International Concern on January 30.)

Medicine also can be slow to give its imprimatur to eminently logical concepts. For instance, we've known for decades that screening colonoscopies detect precancerous polyps, which 30 percent of Americans ultimately develop. And we know that removing these polyps prevents colon cancer. But there was a lag of several years before it was felt established that colonoscopies could prevent death from colon cancer. Not until September 2001, did Medicare start paying for them. (I remember the month because I was delighted that my patients could have colonoscopies, which I'm not trained to do, and I could stop doing flexible sigmoidoscopies, which were a pain in both my and my patient's ass.)

According to the Johns Hopkins website, COVID "may spread through airborne transmission, when tiny droplets remain in the air even after the person with the virus leaves the area."

"Is it possible that there is aerosol transmission?" Dr. Fauci asks. "Yeah, it certainly is."

As with all things COVID, humility is important. But I think the evidence favors aerosols as a mode of transmission. N95s stop aerosols; surgical masks are less reliable.

We need a Manhattan Project to manufacture N95s and distribute them to docs and nurses, policewomen and men, first responders, and TSA employees on the front lines of this war.

Addendum: On September 18, the CDC posted the following:

COVID could be spread through "respiratory droplets or small particles, such as those in aerosols, produced when an infected person coughs, sneezes, sings, talks, or breathes. These particles can be inhaled into the nose, mouth, airways, and lungs and cause infection. This is thought to be the main way the virus spreads." It added, "There is growing evidence that droplets and airborne particles can remain suspended in the air and be breathed in by others beyond six feet (for example, during choir practice, in restaurants, or in fitness classes.) In general, indoor environments without good ventilation increase the risk."

On September 21, possibly responding to political pressure, the CDC removed this guidance from its website.

On July 9, the WHO announced that airborne transmission of COVID in crowded, indoor locations with poor ventilation "cannot be ruled out."

DO ONTO OTHERS

April 2

Speaking of masks...

Before she walks into an operating room, the first thing a surgeon does—before scrubbing her hands and forearms, before backing open the door to the OR and slipping into the sterile gown held out for her by a nurse, before donning sterile gloves—is put on a mask. She does this to prevent any microorganism from contaminating her patient's exposed tissue—whether by the surgeon's cough, spittle, or the mere exhalation of a breath—*not* to protect herself.

Just over a month ago, the U.S. surgeon general, Jerome Adams, tweeted, "Seriously people—STOP BUYING MASKS! They are NOT effective in preventing general public from coronavirus, but if health care providers can't get them to care for sick patients, it puts them and our communities at risk!" The last part of his statement is certainly true, but the first is more complicated.

MIT's Lydia Bourouiba studies how viruses are dispersed through coughs, sneezes, and exhalations. She says, "There's no evidence whatsoever to suggest that surgical masks are *protective* against the smallest droplets"— viruses disseminated as aerosols. Says Harvard epidemiologist Bill Hanage, "I've been slightly dismissive of masks, but I was looking at them the wrong way. You're not wearing them to stop yourself getting infected, but to stop someone else getting infected." And if people are infectious before they get sick, which they are—the CDC now says that a significant percentage of COVID positive persons never develop symptoms, something suggested weeks ago when Iceland extensively tested its citizens—then "everyone should wear a mask in a public space," says Thomas Inglesby of the Johns Hopkins Center for Health Security, "in one additional societal effort to slow the spread of the virus down."

Before walking into a supermarket in Austria, masks are required. In the Czech Republic, anyone in a public space must wear a mask. Everyone wandering the Old Jewish Cemetery or gazing upon the Kafka statue on Dusni Street covers their face.

The Japanese custom of mask-wearing dates to the 1918 flu pandemic, the only time in history Americans wore masks en masse. In 1923, Japan's Great Kanto Earthquake triggered a massive inferno that consumed 600,000 homes. Skies were smoke-filled for weeks, and air quality suffered for months. Masks came out of storage and were common on the streets of Tokyo and Yokohama. A second flu epidemic in 1934 sealed Japan's love affair with the mask. And in the 1950s, rampant air pollution and the unbridled growth of the pollen-rich Japanese cedar tree, which flourished as carbon dioxide levels rose, led to habitual mask wearing. And there's the Japanese custom of courtesy. In normal times, if you see a masked Japanese woman, chances are she has a cold and would be mortified to have infected you.

Regarding mask wearing, the Koreans and Chinese have joined their Japanese neighbors. One reason is philosophical. The three countries are influenced by Taoism and the health precepts of traditional Chinese medicine, in which breath and breathing help determine optimal health. In Chinese cosmology, which overlaps with Chinese physiology, "Qi" is translated as "air" or "atmosphere." When bodily Qi is depleted, or its movement deranged, pain and disease occur; breathing is critical to maintain a healthy Qi.

In Asia, masks don't function as shields. Rather, they're symbols of civic-mindedness, acknowledging that society takes the pandemic seriously, facilitating a we're-all-in-this-together frame-of-mind. Imagine that, in the nation POTUS works so hard to divide!

In China, where masks are mandatory, people comply. South Korea wants everyone to wear masks, though lately, with supplies dwindling, they've had to ration them to two per person each week.

Tragically many Asia-Americans are afraid to wear masks, worrying they'll make others nervous or provoke a racist attack, a risk POTUS's repeated use of the term "Chinese virus" has exacerbated.

Today Eric Garcetti, the mayor of Los Angeles, urged everyone out in public to cover their face. Not with an N95, or even a surgical mask, because they're hard to come by, and because doctors and nurses need them, to turn clinics and hospitals into safer environments for their patients and themselves.

If a perfect world combated COVID, face-covering would be mandated in convenience and grocery stores.

At Mayo, as with all things COVID, counsel on masks has quickly evolved. A week ago today: "All staff who can anticipate direct patient contact (patients within six feet or closer) may begin wearing a facemask throughout their shift" in the hospital.

Needing to grant permission may seem superfluous or even silly. Unfortunately it's not. Dr. Neilly Buckalew was fired from her job in a Boise, Id. hospital when she refused to stop wearing her N95. The administration said if she wore one, others would want them, and there weren't enough. Until recently, Dr. Henry Nikicicz worked as an El Paso anesthesiologist. Anesthesiologists are experts at intubations of the windpipe, an "aerosol-generating procedure" in medical parlance, though talking and breathing, as discussed yesterday, produce aerosols, too. The day after wearing an N95 to intubate a patient, a supervisor told him he could only wear one in the OR or if treating a patient with a confirmed infectious disease. The 60-year-old Nikicicz, who has asthma, responded by saying he was susceptible to respiratory infections. The supervisor texted back, in all caps, that Nikicicz was the only one in the entire hospital wearing an N95 mask and he wouldn't be able to get one when the "real virus" appeared.

The real virus had already arrived, Nikicicz responded. When the doctor kept wearing his specialized mask—think of an N95's fabric as pick-up sticks in miniature, throwing obstacles in the virus's path—he was terminated for "insubordination." According to the University Medical Center of El Paso, he was "told on numerous occasions by his supervisor to not wear the N95 mask while not in the OR or while not treating patients with an infectious disease."

Nurses, too, have been deep-sixed, in more ways than one.

Three days ago, Mayo gave permission for doctors and nurses to wear masks in the clinic setting. Yesterday, the policy became mandatory.

Our inpatient, the only one in the hospital, remains on a ventilator in the ICU.

This morning in huddle, where the internal medicine doctors and nurses teleconference, we were shown a graph depicting when Wisconsin can expect the peak of our surge: April 27. It's projected we'll have enough beds, ICU and in general, to care for the sick.

But the projections cover the entire state. Nearly two-thirds of Wisconsin's 1,730 cases are in Dane and Milwaukee counties, where African-American residents of the latter, like African-Americans in other urban areas, have been especially hard hit (because of past policies such as redlining, blacks in the inner city live closer together than do whites in the suburbs) while southeast Wisconsin has most of the rest. Eau Claire, Chippewa, and Dunn counties have only 28 cases combined, and just that one in the hospital. To be sure, we'll have more cases in western Wisconsin, but in my view we won't see a surge.

Not this spring, at least.

Meanwhile POTUS protégé Ron DeSantis, he of "who me, close our beaches?" fame ("Great governor," POTUS said yesterday) finally bowed to weeks of pressure and reams of scientific evidence and issued a stay-at-home order for Florida, of course exempting churches, which will continue to flout an earlier directive limiting gatherings to ten or less souls, letting them continue infecting their elderly congregants; epidemiologists worry about the ravages COVID will inflict on 4 million-plus 65-and-older Floridians.

POTUS, after a brief flirtation with sanity, like the green flash of a tropical sunset, still refuses pleas for a nationwide lockdown, while simultaneously admitting that our COVID trajectory looks a lot like Italy's: in time, as many as 240,000 American deaths. As he's bowed to the Federalist Society for their blessing of Supreme Court nominees, the I-don't-take-any-responsibility-POTUS, favoring federalism, shirks every chance he's had to lead.

"I trust the states," he says. "Some of them don't have much of a problem."

HOPE, AND SCIENCE

April 3

"It's a game changer," said POTUS of hydroxychloroquine. "A gift from God."

POTUS had teased the drug in his daily press conference ("very exciting") the day before he touted it like Rush Limbaugh hawking a product on his show.

In the study that caught POTUS's eye and short attention span, patients from Marseilles, France, were given azithromycin, a commonly-used antibiotic, and hydroxychloroquine. The researchers looked at laboratory data from the patients and a control group given placebos. Though the lab data seemed promising, clinical outcomes weren't evaluated.

Dr. Jerome Groopman is a Professor of Medicine at Harvard. Among his books is *How Doctors Think*. Groopman lives and works in Boston, where more than 150 hospital workers have contracted COVID. He has relatives in New York and New Jersey who are sick with the virus and fighting for their lives.

Dr. Jean-Michel Molina had worked in Groopman's lab in the 1980s. Molina and his colleagues gave the above drugs to patients in Paris. Results were published three days ago. The cocktail doesn't work.

Outcomes from a Chinese study published the same day are more equivocal. Seventy-eight of 80 patients were deemed to show "clinical improvement." But according to Groopman, careful analysis of the data reveals a "striking finding." Eighty-five percent of the treated patients had no fever, and 92 percent of them were in the lowest category for clinical deterioration. We know that many people infected with the virus have no symptoms at all; an alternative reading of the data, which Groopman finds more plausible, is that the researchers merely observed the natural history of the disease in patients not destined to deteriorate. Groopman cites the hoopla over hydroxychloroquine as a cautionary tale. Physicians—and leaders—must not give false hope.

"Hope is a good thing," Andy told Red in *The Shawshank Redemption.* "Maybe the best of things. And no good thing ever dies." Physicians can, and should, offer hope. Even in a terminal case, there can be hope for less pain, hope for a few more days spent with loved ones. Religious people may look forward to reunions with predeceased friends and family.

In the current pandemic, hope is a precious commodity. We cling to it, as we should, but we must be careful about how it's doled out. Physicians in particular. Honesty and doctoring must be synonymous. Difficult times produce desperate patients, longing for any treatment that might possibly help. Oncologists, and doctors who care for the obese, as can be imagined, need to be especially scrupulous.

Last summer my bride and I had the privilege of a European honeymoon. After a day in Athens, where we visited the Parthenon, we flew to the Greek isle of Kos, birthplace of Hippocrates, the first person to practice scientific medicine. At the ruins of the Asclepeion, the world's first medical school, founded 2,400 years ago by Hippocrates, my eyes grew moist. How humbling to be an heir to his grand tradition!

At the Hippocrates Museum, I bought a keepsake. On the wall of my office, I look up to a framed Oath of Hippocrates, scrolled on faux-parchment and graced with his image. There's even an olive leaf, preserved beneath plastic. "I will follow that system of regimen which according to my ability and judgement I consider for the benefit of my patients and abstain from whatever is deleterious and mischievous."

Before Hippocrates, so-called physicians invoked deities to heal the sick. Back to the future? Please, no.

Antibiotics attack several bacterial sites. Penicillin interferes with cell wall synthesis by shutting down a molecule called peptidoglycan. Vancomycin inhibits this molecule in a different way. Cipro and Levaquin target DNA gyrase, which unwinds DNA for replication, preventing the same. Some antibiotics inhibit the synthesis of RNA, others the formation of folate.

Viruses, because of their simpler structures, are tougher to treat. Most viruses contain only RNA or DNA surrounded by a protein shell, presenting limited targets for potential virucides. The first cases of HIV/AIDS were described in 1981, the year I went to med school, and it took 15 years for scientists to come up with the triple-drug cocktail that's changed HIV from a death sentence to a chronic disease.

Anti-HIV medicines work via several mechanisms. AZT inhibits reverse transcriptase, the enzyme transcribing RNA to DNA—a unique feature of the retrovirus family to which HIV belongs—a step that allows the virus to replicate. Efavirenz attacks the same enzyme but takes a different approach. (The summer after my first year in med school I worked in Howard Temin's lab, washing test tubes and following the dictates of Temin's socially inept grad student. Seven years earlier, in 1975, Temin won the Nobel Prize for his discovery of reverse transcriptase.) Lopinavir and ritonavir are protease inhibitors, which prevent cleavage of polyproteins into the subunits subsequently assembled into the virus's coat.

Because of anecdotal reports of lopinavir and ritonavir helping patients with COVID, and lab data suggesting efficacy, the drugs were put to the test. The study, published recently in the *New England Journal of Medicine*, shows that the drugs have scant if any benefit and potentially serious side effects.

For Hepatitis B and C, it took decades to devise effective treatments that patients could tolerate.

"Yeah, I'm dead right on this," Rush Limbaugh said. "The coronavirus is the common cold." In a sense, he was right. Of seven human coronaviruses, four cause mild illness—the common cold, for which there's still no cure—while the other three, zoonoses that jumped from an animal to one of us, can be lethal: SARS, MERS, and COVID-19. Was Limbaugh so ignorant as to confuse COVID with a benign coronavirus? Or did he know the difference and bury the truth? Which is worse?

Like everyone, I'd love to have a treatment for COVID. But wishing won't make it so. We can't count on a magic bullet to deliver us.

In time, there will be a vaccine. Of this I'm sure. But to distribute it to all in need, plan on at least a year. In the meantime, social distance and wash your hands. Especially social distance.

Because even at a distance, we're together. In the words of Pope Francis delivered a week ago on a rainy day to an empty St. Peter's Square, "Thick darkness has gathered over our squares, our streets, and our cities. We have realized that we are in the same boat, all of us fragile and disoriented, but at the same time important and needed, all of us called to row together, each of us in need of comforting the other."

Peace.

FROM TOO BUSY TO NOTHING TO DO

April 4

Oct. 3, 1988, my first day at the clinic that used to be Midelfort, I saw 13 patients, which turned out to be the fewest I would see on a given day for several years. That first morning, my nurse, Nancy Jevne, who continues (for the most part) to put up with me, walked into my office and took a seat.

"What do you think about generic medicines?" she asked.

I thought for a moment before replying, "They're okay, I guess, except anticonvulsants." (The same drug manufactured by different companies can vary in the amount absorbed, leading to unpredictable drug levels, a potential problem for patients prone to seizures.)

Nancy asked me another question, which I can't remember.

That was my orientation. Two days later, Nancy laid a pile of charge sheets on my desk.

"You have to fill these out," she said.

"Really?" I asked. I thought that someone listened to my dictation, or read its transcription (I surprised myself by learning how to use the Dictaphone all by myself; clinical notes as medical student and resident were written by hand) and decided how much to charge.

"Really," she said, partially concealing an eye roll before walking out.

The day I started my practice, Dr. Terry Borman left the internal medicine department to become Midelfort's medical director. He bequeathed to me a framed Hippocratic Oath that, in turn, had been given to him in 1976 by Dr. Jack Wishart, when Wishart retired and Borman started his career at the clinic. (In his time, Dr. Wishart was a legend; one of the wings of our medical complex is named for him. But when I googled John Wishart, the sole "hit" was the plot of his burial site, in Forest Hill Cemetery, where he was laid to rest 20 years ago.)

In 1995, the Oath moved with me from the Clairemont to the Luther campus and again in 2006 from the west to the east side of the clinic, where it hangs on an exam room wall.

I took Dr. Borman's place in the call schedule, starting with the weekend after my first week on the job. Drs. Shelley, Casper and Spitz handed me their patient lists—Dr. Spitz was kind enough to type his; his handwriting, even for a doctor, was famously, or infamously, indecipherable—and I managed to find my way to the twenty-or-so patients on assorted floors of the hospitals, Sacred Heart first, followed by Luther, where my fourth grade teacher awaited me in the CCU.

I was fairly confident, clinically. I used to say (not anymore) that I was more comfortable treating a patient in cardiogenic shock than one with a rash, because I'd seen the former oftener, but I'll admit to some trepidation about assuming the role of Mrs. R's doc, if only for the weekend. I sat at the nurses' station and studied her chart, memorizing each lab result and reading every clinician's note; as a fourth grader, Mrs. R had had a favorable impression of me, which I didn't want to tarnish. I tracked down her nurse, who gave me the latest scoop: Mrs. R was doing well. I took a breath and walked in her room.

Mrs. R, snow-white hair loosely curled, hospital gown cinched around her neck, opened her arms and exclaimed, "Oh, Steve! Not to worry! The doctor" (Jan Clarke, a cardiologist) "has already been in. But I remember, back in fourth grade, when you were the jack-in-the-box in the school play!"

Usually, the benefits of practicing medicine in your home town outweigh the drawbacks.

Back then, call was every fourth night and every fourth weekend, Friday afternoon through Monday morning at seven. Mondays were my call nights, unless I worked the weekend before (we didn't want to pull four nights in a row) in which case I took call on the following Thursday; every 28 days, I worked 12 days straight, five of them on call.

Busy, but not as busy as residency. In Honolulu, where I served the last two years of my training, I once worked four months without a day off. As an intern in Lexington, Kentucky, I met Melonie, a nurse at the UK Hospital. She became my wife and the devoted mother of our three great kids, Dan, Nicole, and Erik. My year in Kentucky, I worked 20 of 21 days, one day off each third Sunday: laundry day. I had just enough socks and underwear to make it three weeks.

I'm not complaining. On each step of the journey, colleagues shouldered the same load. Together we grew—and continue to grow—in the practice of medicine, a lifelong process, learning to care for the sick.

This earlier life is a fading dream. The medical complex is a shell of its former self. A sign in front of the revolving doors of the clinic entrance declares "No visitors." Employees and patients are screened at the door. "Any coughing or fever or shortness of breath?" Temperatures are taken. If it's above 100.3, you're turned away; we've been told that "a few" employees have tested COVID positive. The pharmacy is barricaded by tables, no patients allowed, while masked pharmacists and techs scurry behind a counter, packaging prescriptions for "drug runners," also masked, who bring them to patients waiting outside in a queue of cars.

Empty hallways converge at the typically bustling patient registration area in the middle of the hospital, staffed by a single lonely receptionist seated behind a desk. If you chance upon someone, they're wearing a mask. It's eerie, a little scary, and also sad.

The internal medicine lobby and its social-distanced chairs are unoccupied. Transparent plastic shields have been erected in front of a solitary greeter (usually, they're a pair) and the sole scheduler, who's typically joined by two colleagues.

There's little for me to do. Thursday I called five patients, and yesterday I phoned six. Not one face-to-face appointment in two days! It's shocking, really. Anyone who doesn't absolutely need to be seen in person is managed by phone or by Zoom, a videoconferencing technology I've yet to, but must, learn. To protect patients and staff, we're minimizing face-to-face contact.

In Eau Claire, we have 14 internists, six at the Clairemont campus and eight at Luther. Starting next week, only one provider will be physically present at each site. Everyone else will work, such as work is, from home.

"There is no historical comparison for what our country is going through," says NYC Mayor Bill de Blasio. "Medically? We're rivaling the 1918 Spanish flu epidemic. Economically? We're seeing unemployment that could look like the Great Depression? Critical supplies? We need to produce more, faster, than any time since World War II."

This time I agree with him, yet on March 13, as the epidemic raged in Westchester County just north of the city, his advice to New Yorkers to "go about their lives" was criminally negligent.

A huge mismatch exists between the supply of doctors and nurses and the need for them in assorted locales. In New York City, in New Orleans, and in Detroit there aren't nearly enough, while places like Eau Claire have too many, at least right now. De Blasio wants to enlist health care workers in a national force to be mobilized to where they're needed most.

This is my generation's World War II. I hope his idea comes to pass.

The CDC now encourages people to cover their faces in public spaces, to make them safer for everyone else. POTUS says, "This is voluntary. You can do it, or you cannot do it. I don't think I'm going to be doing it."

When asked why he himself wasn't following his advice, POTUS said, "I'm feeling good. I just don't want to be doing—somehow sitting in the Oval Office behind that beautiful resolute desk, the great resolute desk, I think wearing a face mask as I greet presidents, prime ministers, dictators, kings, queens, I don't know, somehow I don't see if for myself. I just don't."

On the same day, the White House announced that anyone seeing POTUS or his Vice must submit to a rapid test to prove that they're COVID-free.

PREVENT NOW, OR TREAT LATER

April 5

Midday on Nov. 30, 2006, the eve of World AIDS Day, after a redeye flight from Chicago, I landed at London's Heathrow Airport. Mark Schulz, the lead pastor at Peace Church, and Jill Borgwardt (now Wendtland) accompanied me. We had a few hours to kill before flying to Abuja, en route to Jos, Nigeria, where we'd connect with an AIDS mission sponsored in part by Peace. Mark and Jill (she stayed two years while Mark and I headed home after a week) attended to spiritual education, while I did doctor stuff.

"This way," said Mark, pointing to a staircase up and out of the Underground. Among Mark's many cognitive skills is an inerrant sense of direction, reminiscent of an 18th century Native American scout, which I find all the more impressive as I'm navigationally inept. We emerged onto a five-corner intersection patrolled by an occasional double-decker bus and a swarm of cars driving on the wrong side of the road. My jet-lagged, plunked-down-in-a-strange-city and sleep-deprived self was more disoriented than usual. (With a disquieting frequency, I continue to get lost in our serpentine and sprawling hospital.) As we waited for the pedestrian light, my mind was as hazy as the London sky.

"It's off in this direction," said Mark as we stepped off the curb.

While many London tourists first opt to see Big Ben or Westminster, our destination was the John Snow Pub, on Broad Street, to which, at my urging, Mark guided us. How thrilling to pose for a picture next to a sculpture of the pioneering physician outside of his eponymous pub! But the biggest thrill was yet to come inside the drinking emporium. Behind the bar at which we sipped pints was kept the *actual handle* of the Broad Street pump, the very one that, in 1854, John Snow removed from the pump that provided water to the neighborhood, stopping a cholera epidemic in its tracks. The bartender held out the handle and gently set it in the palm of my hand. The grains of wood, as I caressed a handle smoothed by countless hands through the interceding century and a half, were a palpable thrill.

In the mid-1800s, London's repeated cholera outbreaks were attributed to a "miasma" of polluted air that waxed and waned above the city. During his day, Snow was most famous for giving ether to Queen Elizabeth during her eighth confinement. In addition to his busy practice, Snow was an epidemiologist before the term had been coined. He's considered the father of modern epidemiology—a word derived from "epi" and "demos" that translates into "above the people"—a science of the many.

Snow had studied previous London cholera outbreaks, mapping out the pumps from which victims got their water—most workers at a brewery merely two blocks from the Broad Street pump weren't affected because rather than water they drank beer—a story compellingly told by Steven Johnson in *The Ghost Map*, which I'd read before our trip. Snow traced the source of the Broad Street epidemic to a soiled diaper that contaminated the pump's aquifer.

Sadly, Snow didn't live to see his research vindicated. Even worse, other doctors heaped scorn on him in the four years until he died of a stroke at age 45.

I've seen cholera up close in Port-au-Prince, Haiti, where in the aftermath of the 2010 earthquake I traveled with Mayo medical teams. The bacterium was brought to the country by the UN, which pumped raw sewage into the river that flows through the sprawling slum of 3 million—one of few times in history where a nation has been victimized by an outsider's hygienic misdeeds. In an epidemic that continues to rage, 800,000 Haitians have been sickened and over 10,000 have died.

The disease can kill in a matter of hours. The bacterium triggers a massive secretory diarrhea—electron microscopy video shows the mucous membranes of the small intestine, in a split second, pouring water into the lumen of the bowel like a kitchen faucet turned on full blast—causing victims to lose up to 15 percent of their body weight in a few hours, which without treatment is fatal. One of the most harrowing scenes I've ever witnessed was a ward of 50 infants and toddlers, lying in cribs and tiny beds, IVs in the veins of shaved scalps. Complete silence, no fussing or crying, too sick to make a sound.

It takes time for scientific findings to be disseminated and longer still to apply them. Now as in the 18th century, resistance to science per se is part of the cause. Riots broke out in Liverpool during an 1832 cholera epidemic as protestors accused doctors of poisoning cholera patients and turning them blue. (Cholera has been called the "blue death" because rapid dehydration sometimes leads to slate-colored skin.)

Hamburg's 1873 cholera epidemic prompted city leaders to consider a new sewage drainage system, but for two decades nothing was done. The ruling class viewed environmental pollution not as an offshoot of unbridled capitalism but instead brought on by the dirtiness and unhygienic habits of the lower class. As with the eight red state holdouts against a stay-at-home order to mitigate COVID's ravages, Hamburg had a long history of disregarding medical advice. In 1863, a doctor wrote that the city's rulers had "a scarcely believable ignorance and indifference...to what one may call public health care."

Decades after the introduction of compulsory vaccination for smallpox in the rest of Germany, Hamburg held out, rejecting a plea from the medical profession in 1860 and again in 1871, arguing that mandatory vaccination "encroaches upon personal freedom, and upon the most basic right of the individual, that of the freedom to dispose of his body as he wishes." Later that year, soldiers returning from the Franco-Prussian War carried smallpox home with them, and over 4,000 Hamburg inhabitants died.

And so, in 1892, nearly a decade after Robert Koch's discovery of Vibrio cholerae, the cause of the disease, it was déjà vu all over again. Once more, Hamburg was unprepared for cholera, which killed 8,600 residents.

On Aug. 25 of that year, Koch himself arrived in Hamburg to inspect the city.

"I felt as if I was walking across a battlefield," he wrote. "Everywhere, people who had still been bursting with health a few hours before and had begun the day full of joie de vivre were now lying stretched out in long rows, shot down by invisible bullets, some with the characteristic rigid stare of the cholera victim, others with broken eyes, others already dead: no lamentations were to be heard, only here and there a death rattle."

Late this morning, driving from Altoona to Eau Claire's south side, I passed the fire station on top of State Street hill. Four young EMTs, three men and a woman, stood next to their shiny red truck. Curious about their use of PPE, I spun a U-turn and parked at the convenience store across the street.

They wear a mask for each patient, I was told, upon each of whom they also put on a mask. Any patient with possible COVID symptoms—fever, cough, shortness of breath—and the first responders reach for their N95s.

"Great," I said.

At Mayo, the policy, consistent with counsel from the WHO and the CDC, is a surgical mask, together with a face shield and gown and gloves, provides sufficient protection when caring for a patient with COVID.

A few days ago, Captain Brett Crozier was relieved of command of the USS Roosevelt. One hundred fifty-five crewmembers have tested COVID positive, more than 10 percent of all known cases in the military. The Secretary of the Navy admonished him for copying an email explaining his plight to others outside of his chain of command.

Crozier was worried about his crew. I suspect he was frustrated with the slowness of the Navy's bureaucracy as his concerns made their way up the hierarchy. As Crozier departed the ship, hundreds of sailors, some in uniform and others in civilian attire, repeatedly chanted his name in a hero's sendoff.

Yesterday, POTUS was asked if he agreed with the decision to strip Crozier of his command.

"One hundred percent," he said. "He wrote a letter. That's not appropriate."

Addendum: Later in the day, after I'd posted the above, I was riding my bike—first time this spring!—when it dawned on me that the fire department, being the fire department, wears N95s because they have a ready supply. The other ambulance company in town, run by Mayo, unsurprisingly follows their guidance on masks: the same as the CDC's. But the CDC site has a caveat regarding N95s. Surgical masks, if used with eye protection, gown, and gloves, *in light of the worldwide shortage of N95s* (precise wording and italics mine), protect nurses sufficiently while they care for a patient with COVID. Optimally, in my opinion, to ensure their safety, everyone doing so would wear an N95.

THE IMPORTANCE
OF IMMIGRANTS

April 6

The greatest physician influencers in the United States are immigrants or children of immigrants. By coincidence, those I esteem most are Indian-Americans. Atul Gawande became a staff writer at the *New Yorker* in 1998, when he was a resident surgeon at Harvard. Among his books is *The Checklist Manifesto*, which has improved patient safety in operating rooms across the globe. The best selling *Being Mortal* discusses end-of-life care and features a poignant exposé about his father, who was diagnosed with and died from a rare cancer as Gawande was writing his book. Before he went to med school, Gawande advised Bill Clinton on health care during the 1992 campaign and worked with his wife after Clinton's election; blame Harry and Louise and not the doctor for the failure of Clintoncare. Gawande, who earned an MPH in addition to his M.D. from Harvard Medical School, is a former Rhodes Scholar and the recipient of a MacArthur genius grant. Super impressive, basically.

Two weeks ago, Gawande published an article arguing that the best way to keep doctors and nurses from getting COVID is to go "full Wuhan": everybody double-gowns, wears foot covers, and uses face shields and N95 masks. Unfortunately, he added, there's not enough PPE to do it.

I've heard Gawande speak several times. He refuses introductions, instead choosing to simply step to the lectern and say, "Hi. I'm Atul Gawande."

This humility facilitates his success. In the midst of this pandemic, our leaders must be humble, because steps taken to fight the virus are never enough. COVID moves faster than even a well-led society can react.

Abraham Verghese is Professor of the Theory and Practice of Medicine at Stanford. After earning an MFA in creative writing from the Iowa Writers' Workshop in 1991, Verghese worked for the U.S. Public Health Service in East Tennessee, using the experience to write *My Own Country: A Doctor's Story of a Town and its People in the Age of AIDS*, which won the Lambda Literary Award and was nominated for a National Book Critics' Circle Award. He followed with the novel *Cutting for Stone*, which spent more than two years on the NYT bestseller list. In 2015, a bygone era when presidents bestowed prominent awards upon honorable people, President Obama presented him with the National Humanities Medal.

Verghese is a vocal critic of electronic health records, decrying technology's interposition between patients and the doctors and nurses who, all too often, because of tech's demands, spend more time documenting patient care than caring for patients.

The third of a triumvirate of extraordinary Indian-American physician influencers is Siddhartha Mukherjee, author of the Pulitzer Prize-winning *The Emperor of all Maladies: A Biography of Cancer*, which he penned while doing an oncology fellowship at Columbia. In today's *New Yorker*, Mukherjee writes that we should count COVID's spread within individuals as well as among people.

Instead of the mild or no COVID symptoms typically experienced by millennials, some young health care workers die from it, including Li Wenliang, the 33-year-old Chinese ophthalmologist reprimanded by the government for sounding a COVID alarm. Did he and others, Mukherjee wonders, perish because of high concentrations of the virus they inhaled in a hospital?

Mukherjee offers suggestive evidence from studies of non-COVID viruses. Peak blood concentrations of HIV shortly after infection with the virus can be obtained. The higher the peak, the sooner the patient becomes sick with AIDS. (The time lag between infection and clinical illness may be a decade.) The infectivity of a virus in the herpes family—which includes genital herpes and chicken pox—transmitted from mother to child rises in proportion to the amount of virus shed from the mother's mouth. And in SARS, caused by another coronavirus, higher viral loads in the nose correlate with subsequently worse respiratory disease.

It may be possible, Mukherjee suggests, to inoculate people with a small dose of COVID—the Chinese successfully did something similar with smallpox more than 900 years ago—and thereby provide immunity to the disease.

Any volunteers?

I help out at our local free clinic, where more than 20 percent of our patients speak Spanish, many of whom milk cows. (60 percent of Wisconsin farm workers are foreign-born.) Some work 13 hours a day, four on and one off, rotating shifts, days alternating with nights. (A lady with two young children I met recently, who milks cows in rural Bloomer, had been a physician in El Salvador before immigrating to the United States.) Because of fear of deportation, intensified by periodic appearances of ICE, some patients are afraid to seek care. I try to make them feel welcome, in part by saying I disapprove of POTUS. Mentioning his name along with a frown and stern shake of my head always get this across, no need for the interpreter, and always elicits a smile of gratitude.

"Give me your tired, your poor, your huddled masses yearning to breathe free, the wretched refuse of your teeming shore. Send these, the homeless, tempest-tossed to me."

Through the centuries, generations have heeded this call, forming a melting pot that renews America, making her great all over again. Take note, POTUS: America was, is, and hopefully always will be a nation of immigrants.

THE STOCK MARKET IS NOT THE PANDEMIC

April 7

"This is going to be the hardest and the saddest week of most Americans' lives," said Surgeon General Jerome Adams yesterday. "This is going to be our Pearl Harbor moment, our 9/11 moment, only it's not going to be localized. It's going to be happening all over the country. I want Americans to understand that."

On Wall Street, the Dow surged 1627 points, or 7.7 percent.

Why the disconnect?

On March 30, Jim Cramer, host of CNBC's *Squawk on the Street*, said market short sellers were "betting against science." But Cramer's not a scientist. To be fair, his comment came in the wake of pharmaceutical giant Johnson and Johnson's announcement that they hoped to start clinical trials of a coronavirus vaccine in September. Soon after Cramer's remark, the FDA authorized two rapid-result COVID tests. Abbott Labs uses polymerase chain reaction (PCR) technology on a nasal swab, delivering a positive result in five minutes and a negative one in 13.

In Abbott's test, viral RNA is denatured and reverse transcribed into DNA—the method through which HIV replicates. PCR then amplifies specific and measurable DNA segments. A cutoff value is established, above which is considered positive, below it negative. (No test is 100 percent accurate. A sensitive test has a low cutoff value, while a high cutoff is more specific, which means less likely to be read as positive when the virus isn't there.)

The second quick test, developed by National Bio Green Sciences, measures antibodies in patients' blood. (As of yesterday, a serology test is also available at Mayo-Rochester, though at this point it's not accurate for recent infections.) Yet more positive news came from San Francisco start-up Kinsa Health, which has distributed across America a million networked thermometers priced at $25 each. The thermometers have pointed to COVID hot spots days before upticks in those areas.

Though all of these advances help, none is a game changer. Only an actual cure, unlikely in the coming months, or a vaccine, hopefully available in a year, warrants that moniker.

The market is felt to exemplify the wisdom of crowds, a crowd that, despite the 1,000-plus daily deaths from COVID we can anticipate in the coming weeks, senses we're turning a corner in the COVID fight. "There's light at the end of the tunnel," POTUS says.

We can't social distance forever. At some point, we've got to reopen the United States. But artificial timelines, if unsupported by science, aren't wise. In our race against COVID, the virus is ahead. In order to slay it, we have to follow its lead, and learn from nations like South Korea who've performed better in their COVID response.

Ezekiel Emmanuel, vice provost of global initiatives and professor of medicine at the University of Pennsylvania—he's also Rahm's brother and an Obamacare architect—has laid out a plan:

1. A nationwide shelter-in-place ought to occur over the next eight to 10 weeks. Everyone except essential workers should stay home until June 1.

2. Find out who *really* has the virus—25 to 50 percent of infected patients are asymptomatic—by performing millions and millions of tests. Quarantine everyone infected or believed to be.

3. Deploy thousands of workers from local and state public health agencies to trace *all* contacts of *each* COVID case, using traditional public health tools, social media, and cellphone data. (South Korea can show us how.) Test each contact and isolate anyone who is positive. Hire tens of thousands of COVID detectives for the task.

It's unlikely Dr. Emmanuel's recommendations will be implemented. For starters, sheltering in place for months on end isn't easy, psychologically. POTUS has refused to initiate such an order for a single day, and there's no reason to think he might. Besides, in order to process new information, and use it to change course, you have to believe you've got something to learn.

POTUS doesn't read. He talks to people who share his point-of-view, and he watches Fox News. POTUS got on his can't-let-the-cure-be-worse-than-the-disease bandwagon after fellow former TV personality Larry Kudlow expressed it on Fox.

Fox anchor Laura Ingraham recently lobbied POTUS to keep promoting hydroxychloroquine, and he departed a meeting with her determined to follow through.

"Take it," POTUS said of the drug. "What do you have to lose?"

Two days ago, in his daily misinformation show, he prevented Anthony Fauci from answering a question about whether the doctor shared his belief in the drug. Turns out that Dr. POTUS's interest in Plaquenil (the trade name of hydroxychloroquine made by Sanofi) may be mainly financial. His three family trusts are invested in a mutual fund in which Sanofi is the biggest holding.

When asked about a recent survey of 323 hospitals conducted by the HHS Inspector General that documented disturbing shortages of PPE and equipment and supplies, POTUS lambasted the journalist for asking such a "horrid" question instead of praising his administration's response. When ABC's Jonathan Karl tried to follow up, POTUS tore into him. "You're a disgrace. A third rate reporter. Never gonna make it."

Conservative columnist Max Boot had held out hope that POTUS might merely be America's worst *modern* president, giving him a chance to beat out a smattering of less than laudables including James Buchanan, Andrew Johnson, and Warren Harding. Buchanan, Boot says, because of setting the stage for the Civil War, *had* been POTUS's main rival for W.O.A.T. (worst of all time), the opposite of G.O.A.T.—Lincoln, by acclamation.

However, in all likelihood, the Civil War would have been fought no matter what, Boot says, whereas there was "nothing inevitable about the scale of the disaster we now confront." In the weeks after HHS Secretary Alex Azar alerted him about COVID—before that, at the end of January, U.S. Trade Representative and POTUS toady Peter Navarro circulated a memo warning the White House about the virus—POTUS spoke at eight rallies crammed with fawning *Keep America Great* folk and took extended rides in his golf cart half a dozen times.

"Whatever happens in November," Boot says, POTUS "cannot escape the pitiless judgment of history. Somewhere, a relieved James Buchanan must be smiling."

In western Wisconsin, there continues to be a single hospitalized patient with COVID. In Eau Claire County, only 21 of 895 COVID tests have returned positive. Increasingly, it looks like our local curve will be flat. Stay home, if you can, keep your distance, and cross your fingers!

Yesterday Wisconsin Gov. Tony Evers issued an executive order delaying the state's primary to June, but the State Supreme Court decided along party lines—it's fallacious to think Wisconsin's court elections are non-partisan—to overturn the order. The Republican-controlled legislature joined

GOP judges in insisting the vote must go on, no pauses allowed, pandemic or not.

We stand alone! The only state of 11 to not postpone its April primary! In the Badger State, do Democrats value human life more than supposedly pro-life Republicans?

Whatever, I'm off to vote.

ON LEADERSHIP

April 8

What makes a great leader? A poor one? Are some people born to be leaders? Must effective leaders learn on the fly? What traits and talents are prerequisites?

According to historians, the greatest presidents led us with wisdom and courage through perilous times. George Washington ushered the U.S.A. into existence, standing to his full 6'2" height as he crossed the Delaware. After serving a second term, he declined a third, refusing the coronation desired by many Americans as a second King George. In his farewell address, Washington advised against factions "by which cunning, ambitious, and unprincipled men will be enabled to subvert the power of the people, and to usurp for themselves the reins of government." Notwithstanding "the inferiority of my qualifications and experience in my own eyes" when he became president, Washington thought he'd "contributed towards the organization of the government the best exertions of which a very fallible judgment was capable."

For freeing the slaves and keeping the country from splitting in two, Lincoln paid the ultimate price. It's humbling to visit his memorial and read his Second Inaugural inscribed in big block letters inside the edifice: "Both parties deprecated war, but one of them would make war rather than let the nation survive, and the other would accept war rather than let it perish. And the war came."

People in the north, together with people in the south, "read the same Bible, and pray to the same God; each invokes His aid against the other. It may seem strange that any men should dare to ask a God's assistance in wringing their bread from the sweat of other men's faces, but let us judge not that we be not judged. The prayers of both could not be answered; that of neither has been answered fully. The Almighty has His own purposes." His concluding words have been seared into the American consciousness. Or have they? "With malice toward none, with charity for all, with firmness in the right, as God gives us to see the right, let us strive on to finish the work we are in; to bind up the nation's wounds..."

In the summer of 1921, on a family vacation in Maine, FDR was stricken with a fever and intense pain in his low back and legs. He awoke the next morning not able to walk and was confined to a wheelchair for the rest of his life. Longtime acquaintance Francis Perkins became America's first female cabinet officer, serving as Secretary of Labor for the duration of FDR's presidency. Before his illness, she had an unfavorable impression of his character. "He didn't really like people very much and had a youthful lack of humility, a streak of self-righteousness, and a deafness to the hopes, fears, and aspirations which are the common lot." She said that FDR's illness and subsequent paralysis caused a "spiritual transformation" that "purged the slightly arrogant attitude he had displayed on occasion before he was stricken."

His wife Eleanor put it a bit more diplomatically. "Franklin's illness proved a blessing in disguise, for it gave him strength and courage he had not had before. He had to think out the fundamentals of living and learn the greatest of all lessons—infinite patience and never-ending persistence." Samuel Rosenman, his chief speechwriter while he was governor of New York, noted the "suffering and pain and physical handicap of many years of paralysis intensified his understanding of the problems of those suffering from the pain of hunger and destitution, and deepened his sympathy for those handicapped by poverty and ignorance and suffering from social injustices." FDR, too, was aware of his metamorphosis. "You know," he said, "I was an awfully mean cuss when I first went into politics."

The rest, as they say, is history, which won't be kind to the present-day leaders of New York. Gov. Andrew Cuomo has received justified plaudits for his performances at daily press conferences but unwarranted accolades for his handling of the pandemic, of which 87 percent of his constituents approve. On March 2, the last time his and NYC Mayor Bill de Blasio's ego could be contained in one room, Cuomo said, "Excuse our arrogance as New Yorkers—I speak for the mayor on this one—we think we have the best health care system on the planet right here in New York. So when you're saying what happened in other countries versus what happened here, we don't even think it's going to be as bad as it was in other countries. We have been ahead of this since day one."

On March 5, de Blasio said, "We'll tell you the second we think you should change your behavior." March 13, he said, "We want people to still go on about their lives." Two days later: "If you love your neighborhood bar, go there now, because we don't know what the future may bring." The next morning, knowing gyms would soon be closed, he went to his for one last workout.

San Francisco closed its schools on March 12, when the city had 18 confirmed COVID cases. The day after, when Los Angeles had 40, it did the same. De Blasio was more concerned with the lunches low-income children would miss out on if they weren't in school. Not until three days later, when confirmed cases in NYC topped 300, did the city shut its schools.

At the time, the mayor said he was considering a city-wide shelter-at-home order, but the governor criticized the geographic perimeter as arbitrary and declared that it wouldn't work. On March 19, Cuomo said, "I'm as afraid of the fear and panic as I am of the virus, and I think that the fear is more contagious than the virus right now."

But by the end of the first week in March, while Cuomo was imposing a porous cordon around a cluster of cases that had been linked to a synagogue north of New York City, the metro's infectious disease surveillance system signaled a spike in ERs of influenza-like illnesses. A few days later, the number of police officers calling in sick jumped appreciably. (As of today, one-fifth of the NYPD is out sick, 1,935 officers have tested COVID positive, and ten have died of the disease.)

On March 19, the same day as Cuomo's fear-is-worse-than-COVID quote, Gavin Newsom issued a shelter-at-home order for 40 million Californians, the nation's first of its kind. That day California had 675 cases, New York 4,152. New York state's stay-at-home order didn't go into effect until March 22, when cases topped 15,000.

Because of its population density—27,000 people per square mile live in Manhattan—and because it's a hub for international travel, NYC couldn't emerge from COVID unscathed. But former CDC director Tom Friedan says if New York had been quicker to the draw, 50-80 percent of the lives that will be lost might have been saved.

When Gavin Newsom was a fifth grader, he discovered in his mother's office a stash of papers reporting on his dismal academic performance and describing something called dyslexia. These papers explained, Newsom said, "why everyone else was running into their parents' arms after school and I was stuck in that shack behind the school every Monday, Wednesday, and Friday with four or five other students." Reading aloud was humiliating. He recalls sitting in class "with my heart just sinking and pounding, hoping that period would end and we'd get the hell out of there, and then getting up and starting to read and having everybody in the class laugh."

High school was worse. His grades and self-esteem plummeted, and his SAT score was a "complete disaster." If not for a partial baseball scholarship to Santa Clara University, he might not have gone to college. But he found a passion for political science and worked hard to master the subject matter. In 1995, he volunteered for San Francisco Mayor Willie Brown's campaign, a job he himself would campaign for and win eight years later.

As my wife and I drove home yesterday after voting, Ari Shapiro was interviewing a man on NPR.

Shapiro: Even as you're preparing for the surge of patients, you are lending (500) ventilators to the national stockpile. Are you confident that if your state does have this spike in cases as projected, you will have the resources you need?

Man: I am confident in this respect. What we've been successful at doing in the state of California is bending the curve, buying us time. We're seeing incremental increases (in cases), tragically in the loss of lives...but most importantly, in the context of our planning, the number of people ending up in our hospitals, in our ICUs. When we look at the totality of our ventilators and our inventory and we look at the modeling over the course of the last month and we look forward in the next few weeks, we're confident that we can lend a hand to others in need.

Shapiro: California has tested more than 100,000 people. How many tests do you need to be doing to have an accurate sense of the spread of this disease?

Man: Millions more. We're up to 157,800 total tests as of today. We're going to start significantly increasing our capacity to test—not just the traditional PCR tests, which are swab-based tests, but now with the serology—Stanford finally got approval from the FDA to begin those protocols. So we're going to start seeing significant increases in the testing, and that will help us not only in terms of providing a baseline for community surveillance to really understand the spread and nature of the virus, but also as we begin to process protocols for getting people back into society and back to some semblance of normalcy.

"Who is this guy?" I asked my wife. "Probably the State Director of Public Health." His tone was uninflected, almost flat, the speech of a bureaucrat, albeit one with an impressive grasp of details. But then, in the same gentle yet authoritative voice, he discussed steps that need to be taken to get his state's economy flourishing, once again.

His name? Gavin Newsom.

Yesterday, when POTUS was asked to evaluate how he'd handled the most recent phase of the pandemic, he said, "I couldn't have done it any better."

Our one inpatient with COVID remains on a ventilator in the ICU. For the last week and half, he's been our only hospitalized COVID case.

Leadership and humility—the second abets the first. Nonetheless, I'm going to be bold. In the weeks ahead, continuing into the summer—unless COVID mercifully dwindles to an overdue death—there'll be new infections locally, but we won't see a surge.

RINOS AND CHINOS

April 9

Christian conservatives want China punished. It's not a headline from *The Onion* or *The Borowitz Report*. I shared this with my wife. "They've already *been* punished!" she said. "Hello?!"

"From the time he rode down the escalator at his Tower, Donald Trump made clear there would be a new sheriff in town when it comes to dealing with China." So says Ralph Reed, who in 1991 rose to prominence as the first executive director of the Christian Coalition. "China lied about the genesis of the virus and under-reported their own cases," he continued. "These are actions that cannot be ignored and for which China must be held accountable." (COVID emerged in Wuhan in late December. Given that New York's leaders failed to take appropriate action for two weeks, while each day witnessing COVID advance, the Chinese might be forgiven for not intuiting they were dealing with a novel virus at the outset of the outbreak; they notified POTUS of the issue Jan. 3.)

"The ironic and disgusting thing about China is they get to both create demand and then fulfill demand," said Gary Bauer, referring to America's dependence on China for pharmaceutical supplies. POTUS appointed Bauer, who formerly headed James Dobson's Family Research Council, to the U.S. Commission on International Religious Freedom.

Bauer said, "I think there's a growing acknowledgment in the U.S. and around the world that China's communist rulers are bad actors and, in some way, there has to be some sort of reckoning for all of this." For good measure, he tweeted, "When we find a vaccine, which will happen, the drug company making it better not manufacture it in China, no sane American would take it."

I must be insane.

South Carolina pastor and POTUS buddy Mark Burns wants China to forgive a significant portion of the $1.1 trillion owed it by the United States. He says POTUS "should lead this response and rally other nations who have been greatly affected by the virus to challenge China on a major scale."

Missouri Senator Josh Hawley, a prominent evangelical and POTUS pal, recently opined that Chinese officials have cost the U.S. and other nations "tens of thousands of lives and billions of dollars as a result of its lies." Hawley added, "The Chinese Communist party has done everything it can to hide the origins of the coronavirus epidemic."

In June 2016, Dobson said not-quite-yet POTUS had come "to accept a relationship with Christ" and was now a "baby Christian." Dobson, a Nazarene, is the son, grandson, and great-grandson of Nazarene ministers—nature and nurture, apples and trees—a Protestant denomination emphasizing radical obedience to God that enables "entire sanctification" (a state of perfect love, righteousness, and true holiness that permits the believer's deliverance from the power of sin). It's a nice marriage of arrogance with humility, as I see it, but what is life without irony? (I have exactly one Nazarene acquaintance. He's a great nurse, fine father, and an interesting and accomplished man.)

Dobson, who has a PhD in psychology, may be most famous for his best-selling book *Dare to Discipline*, which extols the supposed virtues of corporal punishment while serving as a field guide to the logistics of spanking. Which are? Take the miscreant to a separate room, pull down his or her britches, and paddle the exposed bottom with a wooden spoon. After pounding the sin out of the sinner, pull your Christian-in-the-making to your chest, verbally express your love, and send the child, with an admonition to sin no more, on their merry way.

Dobson, who once said that former Constitutional Law Professor Barack Obama had "fruitcake ideas" about the Constitution, speaks of the impetus for such disciplinary tactics in his book, hard-won insights borne of a multi-year struggle to force the family dachshund from its favorite perch.

After a (metaphorical) eternity, Dobson thought he'd solved this particular problem, until he returned from a three-day conference and found Siggie (short for Sigmund Freud) ensconced as the new boss of the house. The wiener dog lay on a toilet seat cover—bad dachshund!—strategically positioned, from the canine's perspective, next to a heater.

"When I told Sigmund to leave his warm seat and go to bed," Dobson relates," he "uttered his most threatening growl. I had seen this defiant mood before and knew there was only one way to deal with it."

With the belt, of course. "What developed next is impossible to describe," he says, before describing it. "I fought him up one wall and down the other, with both of us scratching and clawing and growling and swinging the belt." How the dog wrested control of the whipping implement from Dobson he doesn't divulge.

I'm not making this up. How many children raised by fundamentalist parents become contributing members of the creative class? Thank God my folks didn't bring up me in such a manner! If they had, doubtless, you wouldn't be reading this book.

The mutually reinforcing—imagine a klatch of schizophrenics who share the same delusion—and unholy trinity of prominent evangelicals, POTUS, and Fox News has cast a blight on the land. On Fox, Mike Huckabee had his own show. Six weeks ago, on *Fox and Friends*, attempting to outdo his co-religionists in devotion to an orange-haired huckster, Huckabee said POTUS could "personally suck" the coronavirus "out of every one of the 60,000 people in the world" (60,000 COVID patients then, the number exceeds 1.5 million now) "suck it out of their lungs, swim to the bottom of the ocean and spit it out, and he would still be accused of pollution for messing up the ocean."

On Fox, Jerry Falwell, Jr., is a frequent guest, as is Dallas pastor Robert Jeffress, who claims that "God intervened in our election and put Donald Trump in the Oval Office for a great purpose." Last September, again on *Fox and Friends*, Jeffress said that Democrats were impeaching POTUS because he'd committed the unpardonable sin of beating Hillary Clinton.

"If the Democrats are successful in removing the president from office," he said, "I'm afraid it will cause a civil-war-like fracture in this nation from which this country will never heal."

Small wonder that young people are abandoning the church in droves—throwing out the baby Jesus with the bath water—or that, on recent demographic surveys, the fastest-growing group is "religiously unaffiliated."

RINO. Republican in Name Only. Mitt Romney's a RINO, POTUS says, slinging the epithet like an Olympic hammer-thrower, as is any Republican refusing to check both brain and soul at the altar of the Conman-in-Chief. Seldom do his influential evangelical supporters say something with which Christ would agree. Rather than Gospel truths, they repeat POTUS's lies. Not what Jesus would do, but what he would not. Honestly, has Matthew 25 been excised from their Bibles?

CHINOs, I call them. Christians in name only.

Punish China, screams the CHINO choir.

GRIEVING ON
GOOD FRIDAY

April 10

Boris Johnson, POTUS's equal in nativism and science denial, was just discharged from the ICU. Not until researchers at the London School of Hygiene and Tropical Medicine suggested that 500,000 Britons might die if the prime minister kept letting COVID do as it wished did he encourage social distancing. Because of his tardiness, COVID has overwhelmed Britain's NHS, and the country will suffer more death and disease than it would have otherwise. (The same study predicted this laissez-faire approach in America could cause 2.2 million deaths, a figure high enough, it seems, to have caught POTUS's eye.)

Though the virus doesn't discriminate, it preys more on the disadvantaged, people suffering from poverty and subpar health. In this sense, COVID more closely resembles cholera (even though in 1831 alone cholera killed both the philosopher Hegel and the military theorist Clausewitz) than smallpox or the plague.

Densely populated cities with little to no sanitation are cholera's fertile breeding grounds, explaining why it's been devastating in Port-au-Prince, where three million people live packed together. Cholera has sickened 10 percent of Haiti's citizens. Owing to Haiti's dire socioeconomic straits as the most impoverished country in the Western Hemisphere, the disease will be endemic for decades to come.

Today is Good Friday, an apt time to reflect upon suffering, the suffering borne by black Americans throughout our history, a history that has predisposed them to more than their share of COVID-caused illness and death.

Slavery is America's original sin. Every white U.S. citizen, in my opinion, should watch *Twelve Years a Slave*. You'll never look upon slavery, or the descendants of slaves, the same way. *The Warmth of Other Suns*, Isabel Wilkerson's extensively researched and beautifully written book, tells the story of The Great Migration, when 12 million American blacks, starting after World War I and continuing into the 1970s, escaped Jim Crow by heading north.

Passed over for jobs, redlined into tenements, met with violence when they integrated white neighborhoods (Lorraine Hansberry's classic *A Raisin in the Sun* is a good introduction) black Americans couldn't avoid the discrimination from which they'd tried to break free.

A black person who kills a white is 40 times likelier to be sentenced to death than a white who kills a black. Bryan Stevenson's *Just Mercy* and the movie based on the book bring awful American jurisprudence into a horrifying light. In *An American Marriage*, a novel by Tayari Jones, a young black couple faces a similar injustice, which turns their lives upside down.

The more you know, the more you grieve.

A bit of background can help us comprehend the toll COVID has taken and will continue to take on our country's communities of color. In Chicago, 72 percent of fatalities are black Americans, though less than a third of the city is black. "Those numbers take your breath away," says Lori Lightfoot, Chicago's first black female mayor. She adds that the statistics were "among the most shocking things I've seen as mayor."

In Louisiana, 70 percent of fatalities are black, though blacks comprise only a third of the state's inhabitants. Black Americans make up 40 percent of the deaths in Michigan while representing merely 14 percent of its citizens.

According to Rana Awdish, who practices critical care medicine at Detroit's Henry Ford Hospital, "What it means to be hypertensive or diabetic in Detroit" (diabetes and high blood pressure are risk factors for worse COVID outcomes; the former depresses immunity while the reason for the latter isn't clear) "is there is socioeconomic disadvantage, which makes it difficult for patients to access care for chronic conditions, and means—not to overgeneralize—there is often an inability to keep yourself safe."

Protection from COVID means sealing yourself in—easier for Arnold Schwarzenegger chilling in his mansion with his pets than for poorer families with too many people in too small an abode. If you don't have the luxury of working from home but instead must be out and about, staying safe is more challenging; black people are overrepresented in essential service jobs. "We're all seeing cohorts of families coming in," Dr. Awdish says.

Dr. Abdul El-Sayed, a former Detroit health director and public health professor, notes that the first phase of America's epidemic docked in coastal cities—Seattle, San Francisco, Boston, and New York—whose populations were comparatively healthy and young. But COVID has migrated to the country's interior, where "those people with the higher levels of underlying disease, who are most disconnected from institutions, are most vulnerable." El-Sayed notes that Detroit has the highest infant mortality rate of any large city in the United States. "Obviously, a coronavirus infection and a death before the age of one are two very different outcomes," he says. "But, when you work upstream, the things that predict one event predict the other as well."

Milwaukee is sometimes said to be the most segregated city in America. *Evicted: Poverty and Profit in the American City*, Matthew Desmond's Pulitzer Prize-winning book, describes the hardships encountered by black people trying to find safe and affordable housing in Milwaukee, where the discrepancy between black and white life expectancies is a staggering 14 years.

As of this afternoon, Milwaukee County has had 1,575 COVID cases and 77 deaths. A week ago, black people accounted for 22 of the county's 27 fatalities, though less than four of 10 residents of the city are black. There's no reason to think this death disproportion will change in the coming weeks. (Hopefully, it won't be worse yet because of the primary election held three days ago. One hundred eighty polling locations in Milwaukee had been reduced to just five. If you're black, even in 2020, voting can be dangerous.)

Another reason for the Badger State's racial disparity in COVID outcomes can be traced to Scott Walker, our former governor, who refused to accept Medicaid expansion of Obamacare, which made it more difficult for poor Wisconsinites to access needed care. But Walker's influence was yet more pernicious.

According to Alec MacGillis of *The New Republic*, Walker gave voice to a decisive bloc of resentful Milwaukee County suburbanites and their counterparts in neighboring counties, an uncharacteristically conservative (for a metro its size) cohort of white people who inherited a territory bequeathed to them by 1960s white flight and its attendant racial hostilities.

Though I work in Eau Claire, I've seen evidence of this racism firsthand. In 2016, before I met my wife, I dated a restauranteur from Menomonee Falls, a half hour north of Milwaukee. Though crime rates in Menomonee Falls and Eau Claire are similar, "We Back the Badge" and "Support the Police" yards signs were on vivid display on yards in Menomonee Falls (I've never seen one in Eau Claire) and a sign on the Plexiglas guarding a Walgreens pharmacy warned that the safe couldn't be opened for 15 minutes: time enough, a would-be robber would surmise, to summon the police.

This week, until today, I've worked (if you can call it work, there's little to do) from home. I called five patients today and saw three others, my first face-to-face encounters in nine days. As I drove to the clinic, NPR replayed Andrew Cuomo's plea: "I'm asking health care professionals across the country, if you don't have a health care crisis in your community, please come help us in New York now."

Though she had to leave two children at home, Lisa Love joined 28 Georgia nurses to answer the call. Love, who on NPR sounded like a black lady, described the challenges and satisfactions of being able to serve, concluding by saying, "If you can come, come."

But my employer says no.

Good Friday: a good time to be sad.

Addendum: After Labor Day, POTUS went full throttle pro-law enforcement, with its implicit anti-BLM message, doubling down on the tried and true conservative tactic of fear mongering and pitting us against them; support-the-police signs have sprouted in yards like so many weeds in an untended garden.

Second addendum: We now know that diabetes and hypertension, risk factors for vascular disease, are also risk factors, in COVID infection, for inflammation in blood vessels, including those in the lung, contributing to worse COVID outcomes.

WHEN AND HOW
TO REOPEN

April 11

"I'm going to have to make a decision, and I only hope to God that it's the right decision," POTUS says. "Without question it's the biggest decision I've ever had to make."

The decision is when to lift a stay-at-home recommendation and begin to re-open the economy. POTUS's statements are revealing not because of the self-aggrandizing mode that for him is habitual but because they shrink the scope of the issue to a date in time. May 1? June 1? Split the difference?

Looking ahead, the reality of what he needs to do—what's required of effective leadership—is far more complicated. Unfortunately, dealing with complexity isn't POTUS's strength ("Who knew health care could be so complicated?") nor is planning or even looking ahead for a president who impulsively changes course depending upon what a favored Fox host might happen to say.

But let's start by looking at the problem from his simplistic perspective. Next we'll consider the steps to be taken, beginning now, to allow our country to safely reopen, presenting an admittedly pie-in-the-sky view of the presidential leadership of which POTUS has been incapable, which would allow America to navigate, as smoothly as possible, the next phase of her pandemic response.

As I wrote on April 7, Ezekiel Emmanuel led a group from The Center for American Progress and The American Enterprise Institute that targeted June 1 to reopen the economy. Christopher Murray, the director of the Institute for Health Metrics and Evaluation at the University of Washington, whose forecasts for 100,000 to 240,000 American deaths prompted POTUS to relinquish his delusion of packed churches at sunrise tomorrow, agrees with Emmanuel.

"If we were to stop at the national level May 1," he said, "we're seeing a return to almost where we are now sometime in July," adding that there would be a "huge difference" between May 1 and waiting until the end of the month.

But administration officials have said it's unlikely POTUS will extend stay-at-home guidelines past April 30. He's been talking to business leaders, as he should, who've encouraged him to reopen the country as soon as possible. "The longer we stay shut down," says David McIntosh, the president of the Club for Growth, "the worse off people will be and the harder it will be getting the economy going again and getting people jobs so they can go back to work."

"You know what?" POTUS asks. "Staying at home leads to death also. It's very traumatic for the country."

But it's a false choice to trade public health off against the economy. People, whether they work in "essential" sectors or not (aren't all workers, except maybe stock day-traders, essential?) must be protected on the job, made to feel safe; if you don't feel safe on the job, you won't go to work. Grocers are hiring, but why risk your life for $2/hour in additional hazard pay? Wiser to ride the recession out.

Grocery stores have been slow to set up sneeze-guard partitions at checkout counters and allow workers who so desire to wear masks; many have been sickened, and some have died. Walmart has lost at least two employees to COVID. (Farther up the food chain, COVID has caused closures of slaughterhouses across Colorado, Iowa, Nebraska, and Pennsylvania, where hundreds working elbow-to-elbow have contracted the disease.)

To make grocery stores, pharmacies, and other retail outlets safe for employees and shoppers, everyone should be *required* to wear a mask. (The same rule ought to apply to any business wherein social distancing can't safely occur.)

It's a secret to Asia's success. When you walk into a Chinese or South Korean grocery store, everyone is masked. Rather than saying, "It's voluntary. You can do it; you cannot do it," POTUS should use his bully pulpit (a bully knows how) to mandate the practice. Covering your face with anything less than an N95 might not keep you from contracting COVID, but it'll protect everyone else, an all-for-one and one-for-all mentality (is POTUS capable of such a mindset?) that would not only make everyone safer but instill in each American a sense of shared purpose in the battle against this terrible scourge. Can a man whose first words as president described "American carnage" rise to the occasion and truly inspire? POTUS supporters, what do you think?

Inspiration and policy go hand in hand. As advocated on April 1, make more masks! As women flooded factories during World War II to manufacture the munitions that defeated the Third Reich, conscript the unemployed to churn out billions of masks, both surgical and N95s, to fight the virus.

"Staying at home leads to death, too," POTUS says. This is worth a closer look. Does it, really?

Anne Case is an emeritus professor at Princeton and the author, with Angus Deaton, her husband and fellow economist, of *Deaths of Despair and the Future of Capitalism.* According to Case, fewer people died during the Great Depression of the 1930s than during the roaring 1920s. And during the Great Recession of 2008-9, though a third of Greeks and Spaniards were out of work, their mortality fell.

In boom times, more people are killed in car crashes and on construction sites. There's more air pollution, which affects children and people with asthma, and the elderly get less care. The diseases of despair Case and her husband have described—alcoholism, opioid addiction, and depression—typically take years to cause death.

Which is not to say that the country can be shut down indefinitely. In just three weeks, we've already lost nearly 17 million jobs. But besides producing billions of masks for wide use, how do we safely reopen America?

Test, trace, and isolate. When the country comes back online, few people will have been exposed to the virus. Former FDA Administrator Scott Gottlieb, who served POTUS from May 2017 until a year ago, thinks just 1-5 percent of the country has COVID immunity. (On average; the figure is higher in New York City than in rural Wyoming.) Dr. Gottlieb, now a fellow at the American Enterprise Institute, notes that, in a normal week, patients visit primary care providers 3.8 million times. Strive to test everyone, he says. 750,000 people/day.

POTUS has a different take. "You don't need full testing," he says, merely concentrated screening in hot spots. Yesterday, he said that even without widespread testing COVID "will soon be in full retreat." He'll know, he says, because "people aren't going to go to the hospital, people aren't going to get sick. You're gonna see nobody's gonna be getting sick anymore," he continued. "It will be gone and it won't be much longer."

Good to know.

If POTUS comes to his senses (is it delusional to plead for an Easter miracle?) and puts the full power of the federal government behind a test, trace, and isolate imperative, cases will have to be quarantined and their contacts traced and isolated, too.

Apple and Google announced a new app yesterday that will alert smartphone users when they might have come into contact with a COVID case. The companies hope to publicly release the tool "in the coming months."

South Korea has successfully used similar technology since the start of their epidemic; the first COVID case in both the U.S. and South Korea was January 20; South Korea suffered a worse initial outbreak, linked to the church in Daegu, than did the United States. As of noon today, there have been 211 COVID fatalities in South Korea while American deaths have surged past 20,000. South Korea tests, traces, and isolates with religious zeal.

When COVID hit Wuhan, the Chinese deployed an army of 90,000 public health workers. When the virus attacked New York City, a platoon of 50 had to suffice. Though public health has never been a priority in America, it's not impossible to turn things around.

Sanjay Gupta—at the front of the line when God handed out talents, ladies, don't you think?—says America needs an added 300,000 workers to fulfill this crucial mission, but don't expect POTUS to support the idea the same way his besotted followers, in this crisis, rally around him. When he was asked yesterday what metrics he'd use to decide when to relax social distancing, POTUS pointed to his head and said, "The metric is right here. That's my metrics. That's all I can do."

More self-awareness than his usual, maybe, though instead of pointing to his head, POTUS should have glanced down, placed a palm on his ample paunch, and given it a pat.

EASTER HOPE

Father Rick Frechette is the most impressive human being with whom I've ever had the privilege to work. After studying math and philosophy in college, he went to seminary and, in 1979, was ordained as a priest. While serving a Baltimore parish, he met Father William Wasson, founder of Nuestros Pequenos Hermanos (NPH: Our Little Brothers and Sisters), and went to work at a Mexican orphanage, and then he was sent to Honduras to establish a second orphanage for NPH.

In 1987, Mother Teresa's Sisters of Charity in Haiti gave Father Rick his next opportunity. The sisters were caring for babies of mothers who were dying from AIDS. Many babies died, too, but the survivors needed care. He moved to Port-au-Prince and founded a children's hospice and an orphanage.

Malaria, cholera, dengue fever, chikungunya, leptospirosis, tuberculosis, and HIV are endemic in Haiti. At 64 years, life expectancy in the country is the worst in the Western Hemisphere. Father Rick saw the need—Haiti has one doctor for every 15,000 people while in the United States the ratio is 1:500—and went to medical school, flying back and forth to Haiti while he did, graduating in 1998 from the New York College of Osteopathic Medicine.

In Port-au-Prince, land was purchased for a hospital in Nov. 2002, and construction began the next summer. It took three years plus—the two-story structure was built by hand because heavy equipment wasn't available—and a mere $5 million dollars for the 224-bed St. Damien's Hospital, named for the priest who died while ministering to people with leprosy on Molokai, to become a reality.

It's a beautiful facility, by far the best pediatric hospital in Haiti, an isle of tranquility amidst the chaotic sea of Port-au-Prince. In the courtyard, shrubs and flowers encircle the lawn—rare green space in a country wracked by poverty, its mountains scarred, denuded of trees—and there's a mural of St. Damien, children at his feet. Each year, the hospital cares for 80,000 children and adults.

On the grounds stands St. Philomena Chapel, hewn of hand-cut stone, named after the church on Molokai built by St. Damien. Through stain-glass windows, the sun shines on a brown tile floor. Behind the altar is a mural depicting seven Haitians: two pairs and a grouping of three. All hold hands, in each scene. To the right, an older child reaches down to help a younger child scale a pile of rubble. A single horseshoe-shaped bench lines the periphery of the little sanctuary, to make room for bodies on stretchers to be laid on the floor before the start of 7 a.m. Mass.

One morning three adult bodies borne on handheld stretchers were carried into the chapel. The workers walked out and returned moments later with another stretcher on which I counted 17 small garbage bags. At first, it didn't hit me that each bag held a baby's body.

On January 12, 2010, Haiti suffered a magnitude 7 earthquake. According to a study from the University of Michigan, 160,000 people died. Father Rick, yet again, expanded the scope of his mission, cobbling together from 40' x 12' shipping containers a hospital in which to treat injured adults.

One evening, as I worked in that hospital, now called St. Luc's, Father Rick, drenched from head to toe, carried a convulsing man in his arms. He laid the young man on a gurney, which we faced each other across, yelling to be heard above the din of the monsoon pounding the steel roof like a thousand ball peen hammers.

Father Rick speaks six languages. He's ruggedly handsome—a Sanjay Gupta-esque Italian-American, 66 years old going on 50—with a full head of black, silver-flecked hair. He delivers his homilies in a clerical robe and mud-splattered sneakers.

Some of the sermons have lodged in my brain. Before Jesus preached the Sermon on the Mount, the priest said, he made sure everyone had a comfortable place to sit and enough food to eat. Another homily: the facial muscles used in both crying and smiling are the same; out of tears, given time, joy may arise.

On Maundy Thursday, his Easter blessing showed up in my inbox:

Ecstasy and Agony, in One Holy Narrative.

The palms on the altar also grow in front of the church. They are at our front door.

In the same way, the agony and ecstasy are at your front door, and ours.

The agony is all too terrible, heavy, sad, tragic.

The ecstasy is evident in so much heroism to help suffering and marginalized people, in so much courage and strength and prayer.

We had our first death at St. Luc's today from the infamous Covid-19. We hold up in prayer all who have died in these days.

Be assured we hold you close in prayer, especially during these most holy days.

Praying for a fast end to the pandemic, for your safety, for your strength in distress and in grief, I send our love, prayers and a bear hug.

With gratitude,
Father Rick Frechette

Rick Warren may be the most influential pastor in America. Saddleback Church, which he and his wife started 40 years ago, now claims 180,000 members on four continents. Warren's *Purpose Driven Life* has been translated into 85 languages and has sold 32 million copies. He's trained over a million pastors to guide their congregations by its principles.

Warren, whose son took his life after a long struggle with mental illness, was recently asked, "Where is God in this pandemic?"

He responded by asking, "Where was God when my son died?" After a pause, Warren said, "He's in the same place he was when *His* son died, on the cross. He was grieving the inhumanity of man to each other. He was grieving—the Bible says God weeps. But you also see God in the goodness of people. All these people you see out there helping others, that's God in their hearts."

When Argentine priest Jorge Mario Bergoglio became pope, he chose the name Francis, after St. Francis of Assisi, who died in the 13th century. "Your God is of your flesh," St. Francis had preached. "He lives in your nearest neighbor, in every man."

Last year, Pope Francis delivered his Easter homily to a packed St. Peter's Square. Today, it was nearly empty. Addressing "a world already faced with epochal challenges and now oppressed by a pandemic severely testing our whole human family," Francis encouraged "a contagion of hope." He acknowledged "an Easter of solitude lived amid the sorrow and hardship that the pandemic is causing, from physical suffering to economic difficulties."

"This is not a time for indifference," he continued, "because the whole world is suffering and needs to be united in facing the pandemic." Francis said that "indifference, self-centered-ness, division and forgetfulness are not words we want to hear at this time. We want to ban these words forever."

Francis implored Christ to "dispel the darkness of our suffering humanity and lead us into the light of His glorious day, a day that knows no end."

"Happy Easter," the pope said.

Peace and power.

PANDEMICS, POWER, AND SNAKE OIL

April 13

The first century Roman emperor Nero, who became ruler at age 16, was a disreputable dude. His mother tried to rule by proxy through her son. Five years into his reign, he staged a shipwreck in which she was drowned.

Nero divorced his first wife, Claudia, when he impregnated his girlfriend Poppaea, who he married 12 days after the divorce. During Poppaea's next pregnancy, Nero killed her in a fit of rage by stomping on her abdomen. Statilia, who was married to another man, was Nero's mistress. After the murder, Statilia's husband was forced to commit suicide so she could marry the emperor. Later that year, Nero also married a boy named Sporus and had him castrated. He forced Sporus to appear in public as his wife, dressed in the regalia of Roman empresses.

When an epidemic of bubonic plague killed thousands of Romans, Nero ordered his chief physician to circulate an old miracle cure. "It was an attempt by Nero to sustain his legitimacy in the midst of this catastrophic event," said Aaron Shakow, a medical historian at Harvard, who added, "Epidemics are dangerous to rulers."

This year, in early March, a group of French scientists launched an experiment to see if the 85-year-old drug hydroxychloroquine could be the miracle cure for COVID that everyone sought. Before the study was published online, a lawyer falsely claiming an affiliation with Stanford University appeared on Fox News' *Tucker Carlson Tonight* to tout the results: a "100 percent cure rate against coronavirus." The next day POTUS was hailing the drug as a "game changer" and "a gift from God." The only problem? The study's results failed to match the hype.

The gold standard for a clinical study is the double-blind trial, in which neither patients nor researchers know which treatment is given—placebo or active drug. Patients are randomized into two groups, the baseline characteristics of each made as equivalent as possible.

But in the French study, the treatment and control (placebo) groups came from different populations, the former from the researchers' Marseille hospital and the latter from other facilities in the south of France. Moreover, the study was "open label," meaning both patients and researchers knew which treatment was being administered. The study included just 42 patients, three of whom were transferred to the ICU, a fourth died, one stopped treatment because of nausea, while a sixth left the hospital and was lost to follow up.

If you'd only heard about the "100 percent cure rate" promoted on Fox News, you'd assume the four patients with worse clinical outcomes (three ICU transfers and one death) had been unlucky enough not to receive the "cure." But all four patients, and the two others cited above, were given hydroxychloroquine.

The six patients were excluded from analysis because of how the researchers reported the results: whether or not COVID was present in nasal swab specimens obtained on each day of the study. (Why specimens weren't taken from ICU patients isn't clear.) Based on the swabs of the 36 analyzable patients, the ones receiving hydroxychloroquine cleared COVID from their noses a bit faster than those who didn't.

In summary, an experiment in which 15 percent of the treatment group and no one in the control group had poor clinical outcomes was reported as having a "100 percent cure rate." On April 3, two weeks after the study's publication online, the International Society of Antimicrobial Chemotherapy—itself an obscure organization—publishers of the French study, said the group's board "believes the article does not meet the Society's expected standards."

Didier Raoult, the lead author of the French study, and Harold Bornstein, POTUS's former physician, who'd said that POTUS's "physical strength and stamina are extraordinary" and that POTUS, "if elected, will be the healthiest individual ever elected to the presidency"—bear a striking resemblance. Though probably a coincidence, perhaps POTUS takes a shine to docs with a certain look. Central casting!

Rather than admitting his mistake, Tucker Carlson and his Fox co-conspirators, in typical POTUS fashion, doubled down. "It's probably the most shameful thing I, as someone who has done this for 20 years, has ever seen," Carlson proclaimed last week. "It's making a lot of us ashamed to work in the same profession as those people. So reckless and wrong in the middle of a pandemic, it really is, for real."

The objects of his scorn? "Members of the media" who've criticized POTUS for promoting hydroxychloroquine. Sean Hannity is also mad, hornet-like. (From the movie *Bombshell*: "If it pisses off your grandfather and scares your grandmother, it's a Fox News story.") The drug is showing signs of success, Hannity said, "in spite of what the mob and the media is telling you."

The manufactured controversy about the efficacy of hydroxychloroquine is the most recent variation on Fox's theme of conjuring new culture wars like rabbits from a magician's hat. The strategy works.

In 2005, Bill O'Reilly introduced America to the "War on Christmas," which he opined was being waged from within. At the time, a Gallup poll showed 41 percent of respondents preferred "Happy Holidays" and 56 percent "Merry Christmas." At the end of each year, as the country became more religiously diverse, the network revisited the non-issue. A decade later, only 25 percent preferred "Happy Holidays," while 65 percent chose "Merry Christmas."

On Fox, the enemies conceived (POTUS's lifeblood) are often elites portrayed as opposing that which the loyal viewership knows to be righteous and true. On her program April 9, Laura Ingraham said, "After hearing all of the stories where hydroxychloroquine is credited with saving lives, it is amazing that the left and the medical establishment is still in total denial about the potential of these decades-old drugs."

Earlier, Fox weekend host Jesse Watters denounced the "cherry-picking snakes, liars and backstabbing hypocrites" who've prevented patients from receiving hydroxychloroquine. "The president was hopeful but was savagely attacked in the media," he said. As an example, he played a clip of Rachel Maddow calling POTUS's hype "cruel and harmful...and wildly irresponsible from anyone in a leadership role," which sounds accurate to me.

According to Dan Cassino, a political scientist and author of *Fox News and American Politics: How One Channel Shapes American Politics and Society*, "Even if there's not a lot of disagreement in the medical community about the use of hydroxychloroquine, the fact that you can point to people on both sides means that any opinion is justified."

Voila, controversy.

Rupert Murdoch's misinformation machine isn't limited to Fox News. What was Jerry Hall thinking? I used to think she was cool! Murdoch's *Wall Street Journal* has jumped on the hydroxychloroquine bandwagon, cheerleading the drug in two recent editorials.

People who've studied POTUS's tweets say that the more outrageous, the more demonstrably false, the more frequently re-tweeted are the Conman-in-chief's missives. Counterintuitive though it seems, P.T. Barnum understood.

Before and after the 2016 election, I asked dozens of patients their political opinions. Every POTUS supporter watched Fox, and none solicited my perspective. (Maybe the majority already knew.)

In the field of psychology, the Dunning-Kruger effect is a cognitive bias in which people with low aptitude at a given task overestimate their ability. My personal take is Dunning and Kruger were half right. No one's immune to inappropriate cockiness. Like COVID, the tendency doesn't discriminate, based on IQ or anything else; according to a classic study, more than 90 percent of college professors thought themselves "above average."

Isaac Asimov may have said it best. "There is a cult of ignorance in the United States, and there always has been. The strain of anti-intellectualism has been a constant thread winding its way through our political and cultural life, nurtured by the false notion that democracy means that my ignorance is just as good as your knowledge."

So it's no surprise that at Anthony Fauci, POTUS is pissed.

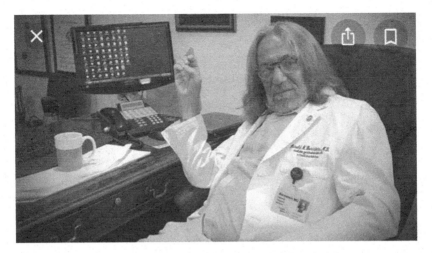

Harold Bornstein, M.D.

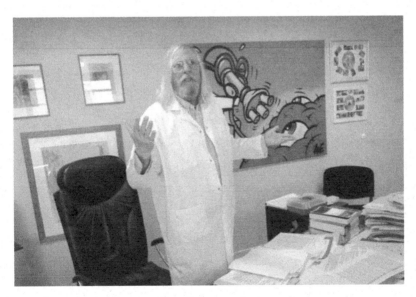

Didier Raoult

THE PLEASURES
AND PITFALLS
OF UNCERTAINTY

April 14

COVID was identified little more than three months ago. Every day we learn more, as doctors and scientists around the world race to develop treatments and vaccines, but there's much we still don't know.

Starting with immunity. In 1846, during a measles outbreak, the Danish physician Peter Panum visited the Faroe Islands (between Scotland and Iceland) and made a seminal observation: residents born before a 1781 outbreak were immune to getting measles again, the first demonstration of lifelong immunity to an infectious disease.

Immunity to coronaviruses is more complicated. According to Mark Lipsitch, the director of Harvard's Center for Communicable Disease Dynamics, definitive information on the topic is not yet available. Antibodies to SARS and MERS, COVID's closest cousins, persist in the blood for two to three years, though they wane over time. Another data point: when healthy volunteers were inoculated with a benign coronavirus that causes colds, they retained some resistance to similar bugs a year later.

Most patients infected with COVID develop antibodies, but it's not clear how protective they are. Of 175 Chinese patients with mild symptoms from the virus, 70 percent had a strong antibody response, 25 percent a weaker one, while 5 percent had none at all.

Lipsitch guesses that most patients infected with COVID will be immune to it for "a year or so."

More uncertainty. Documented U.S. COVID cases now exceed 600,000, but the actual number, though unknown, is higher. How much? A consensus is a factor of 10, though some scientists think the number could be higher yet by another order of magnitude. Supporting this perspective, according to an article published yesterday in the *New England Journal of Medicine*, 15 percent of *asymptomatic* NYC women presenting to hospital for childbirth were COVID positive.

Determining the prevalence of current and former infections across the country will tell us when herd immunity can offer some protection from the virus. For measles, which is very contagious, more than 90 percent of a population must be immune for the herd to be able to protect. For herd immunity against COVID, which is three times more transmissible than the flu but five times *less* infectious than measles, 60 percent of a population must be immune. Herd immunity to COVID will be established, if it is, quicker in NYC than it will be in northern Wisconsin.

We simply don't know, Dr. Lipsitch says, without extensive testing, how many people across the country have contracted COVID.

If doctors and researchers admit areas of ignorance, think of the predicament for citizens and politicians!

Except POTUS. Yesterday, during his daily press conference, arguably his most deranged performance yet, when asked about a NYT exposé that detailed, over the last two and a half months, his many failures to behave as any normal leader would, POTUS responded, "Everything we did was right." The rest of the performance, after a propaganda video, consisted of a tirade against the questioning journalists. How can a leader lead when he constantly craves ego strokes and lambasts anyone who doesn't comply?

In dramatic contrast with last week's paean to federalism—pivoting to dictatorship faster than you can say "I don't take any responsibility at all"—POTUS now says *he* calls the shots about how and when to reopen the economy. "When you're the President of the United States, your authority is total!"

Of course, like much of the drivel that spills from his mouth, this ain't true. What's he gonna do? Force old Mrs. Jones in Tuscaloosa to stay in her home, when he wouldn't make her earlier? Fortunately, POTUS is becoming irrelevant. He'll always be King Lear, but the nation's governors, with responsibility for the pandemic placed by default in their more capable hands, refuse to be led as if blind.

I myself will pivot back to uncertainty.

On March 15, Dr. Fauci said, "I think we should really be overly aggressive and get criticized for overreacting." Four weeks later, on Easter Sunday, he said, "I mean, obviously, you could logically say that if you had a process that was ongoing and you started mitigation earlier, you could have saved lives. Obviously, no one is going to deny that." In other words, America did the opposite of overreact.

But in a pandemic, what does it mean to overreact? How do you know, in real time, if a given act, or a specific directive, is excessive? Even in hindsight, how to sort this out? But because COVID infects people faster than they can sort out how to handle it, some overreaction appears wise.

Honestly, though, why aren't there any eggs or TP on the grocery store shelf? Part of the reason, suggests risk-communications consultant Peter Sandman, is that doing *something* distracts the brain, letting a man, for instance, shake off his paralysis and get off the couch. After all, COVID is a novel virus. How can we know for sure how to react?

Facing this conundrum, uncertainty allies with panic. "Our guts are way ahead of our understanding," Sandman says. And if you consider the four horseman of the apocalypse—Death, War, Famine, and Pestilence—it's the last we worry least about.

The less we think, the more we join the herd. I needed gas on the evening of 9/11 and was surprised to find a long line of cars that had beaten me to the neighborhood convenience store.

Some are comforted, apparently, by communitarian retail sprees like Black Friday's, though don't take it from me, because other than at bookstores, my opinion is that shopping sucks.

Could there be a strange and to me indecipherable logic to descending en masse upon retail purveyors of consumer goods? What's the downside to extra diapers or disinfectant wipes? You're preparing, exerting control.

"Many people hold the implicit belief that big problems require big solutions," says Steven Taylor, author of *The Psychology of Pandemics*. "Yet they were told that the big problem should be addressed with small, seemingly trivial solutions, e.g. hand washing. So many people felt that they needed to do more to keep themselves and their families safe. Hence, the excessive shopping."

Still seems weird to me.

As does removing your shoes before you walk in the house. Or wiping clean each piece of mail before you do the same. Or prohibiting golf, though I'm a duffer, and partly for this reason hit the links, and sometimes my ball, infrequently. Sixty-five thousand petitioners haven't convinced Gov. Tony Evers to let Wisconsinites golf. Good grief! Limit riders to one a cart. Better yet, make everyone walk. If you're still paranoid, play without pins, unclear though it is that they can function as disease vectors.

Overreaction, I think. COVID is a *respiratory* virus. Though theoretically possible to contract the virus by touching contaminated surfaces and then your eyes, nose, or mouth, it's far more likely, in my view, to become infected by inhaling a viral aerosol. Over 2,800 members of the NYPD haven't gotten COVID from physical contact with infected citizens but rather from being breathed or coughed upon.

We now have two patients with COVID in our hospital, but no Eau Claire County resident has had a new infection with the virus in more than a week. In my humble opinion, we could reopen our clinic, now in its fourth week of shutdown. Monitor the temperatures of doctors and nurses and patients, make everyone wear a mask—this practice began yesterday— have doctors and nurses wear gloves for each patient visit, and disinfectant surfaces before a new patient is roomed. That's how South Korean has kept their clinics open.

While local doctors' and dentists' offices are shuttered, some chiropractors in Eau Claire have stayed open, neither they nor their patients masked. Are they being irresponsible, are doctors and dentists overreacting, or is the truth somewhere in between?

P.S. Happy 90th birthday, mother!

Addendum: As of February, 2021, according to conventional wisdom, most people infected with COVID have three months of immunity to subsequent infection with the virus.

WILL IT MATTER?
(A SHORT STORY INSPIRED
BY CURRENT EVENTS)

April 15

On the corner of 50th and Fifth Avenue, close to the eponymous Saks, a young teenager named Dominica, black pony tail emerging from a ball cap, waved a copy of the *New York News* above her head. Her father, a cop in Queens, had contracted COVID and was on a ventilator in Lenox Hill Hospital, where her mother worked as a nurse. Before her dad had taken sick, both parents had given their tacit permission (Dominica was a spirited child, with an entrepreneurial streak) for her to sell newspapers in Manhattan, as long as she was home by eight for online instruction at P.S. 78.

After her dad was admitted to the ICU, Dominica was grateful for the job. She worried about him constantly, but being out on the street, compared to staring at her computer at home, Dominica obsessed about him a little less. Fortunately, he was improving. Her mother said they were weaning him from the ventilator. She couldn't wait to see him; in the hospital, no visitors were allowed. Not even family. Her mother, who worked on a different unit, had to plead with her supervisor, a former Army nurse, to enter his room.

This morning at six, there was a peach-colored glow on the eastern horizon, toward which faced her family's fourth-floor walkup, three blocks beyond the East River in Queens. Dominica and her mother walked out of the unit together to start their shifts. "Keep your mask on!" her mother said.

For Dominica, business was slow. Usually, the street would be jammed with vehicles and the sidewalk packed with pedestrians. But not a single yellow cab cruised the street. A rare car sped to its destination like the ambulances whose sirens wailed day and night. Not only were people scarce, they moved slower, as if reflecting unhurried thoughts, less preoccupied now with their next meeting or sale. Everyone acknowledged Dominica. Smiles, hellos, waves of the hand.

A young black man approached. He wore a business suit tailored to fit his athletic physique. His full beard was neatly trimmed, no mask to conceal it. Like Michael B. Jordan but with better facial hair, Dominica thought. He caught her eye, there was a twinkle in his. Or was it a leer? She'd just turned 17. Lately, for the first time, the looks she got made her feel like a woman. Exciting, but also a little scary.

"Hey, sweetness," the man said, stopping in front of her, inside of the safe six-foot range. Dominica smelled his cologne. The surgical mask her mom had pilfered from the hospital felt flimsy, insufficient. Her heart started to throb in her throat. She was aware of her breathing, in and out through the mask, poofed out when she exhaled, brushing her lips when she breathed in. "Whatcha selling?"

"Um," Dominica said. "Just a newspaper."

"Never say *just*," the man said. "*You're* never just a "just," and anything you're selling, it isn't either."

Dominica nodded.

"How much?"

"How much?" she repeated.

"For the newspaper?"

"Three dollars."

He handed her a ten, and Dominica gave him a newspaper, felt in her waist pack for the change.

The man shook his head and said, "Keep it." Before turning to go, he smiled and added, "Stay safe!"

Dominica sold 18 papers. *The News* paid her $15 an hour, and she could count a full hour each hour she worked at least half of, plus a $1 per paper bonus; in an hour and thirty-seven minutes, she'd get $48, not including tips, which this morning came to $21. Michael B. Jordan's $7 tied her biggest yet.

By the time Dominica got off the subway and walked home, she was 15 minutes late. No big deal. Compared to COVID-19, and the classic novels she read for fun, school was boring. Especially first hour. Mr. Smith didn't exactly inspire, nor was geometry fascinating, though she was pulling a high A, same as in every class. She could flunk the remaining tests—she wouldn't, but she could—and still get an A. She muted Mr. Smith's voice on the computer, grabbed the newspaper, opened the sliding door, and walked out on the balcony.

The thermostat said 43 degrees, but the sun, a yellow hot-air balloon hovering above the neighboring buildings, like hers several stories high, made it seem warmer. She unzipped her down jacket. A siren trailed off, like a fading cry for help. From a window below, a pleasing aroma wafted up. Mrs. Rodriguez was making breakfast burritos

Each night at eight, she joined her neighbors on the balcony as they chanted and cheered, rang bells and tooted horns, for the doctors and nurses, nurses like her mom, who took care of the sick, patients like her dad. She'd pounded a pan with a spoon with such ferocity—applauding her mother, willing her father home—that the dents she'd made at first now had dents of their own. She sat down and turned to the paper.

"President Defunds World Health Organization in Pandemic!"

Had to be a mistake. Perhaps the typesetter had forgotten a word or two. Or he'd misunderstood. Probably, he'd meant to say, "President Increases Funding for the World Health Organization in Pandemic." A sane decision, no explanation mark necessary.

"The President announced Tuesday he is halting funding to the World Health Organization while a review is conducted."

Dominica shook her head. There'd been no mistake.

"The President said the review would cover the WHO's role in severely mismanaging and covering up the spread of the virus. Had the WHO done its job to get medical experts into China to objectively assess the situation on the ground and to call out China's lack of transparency, the outbreak could have been contained at its source with very little death."

An intelligent young woman, Dominica knew to not believe anything the President said. Still, there had to be a way to decipher if his words had even a peripheral connection with a kernel of truth.

Like Dominica, her mother had been a straight-A student, double majoring in pre-med and microbiology—until she got pregnant with Dominica, when she switched to nursing. Dominica knew it wasn't her fault, but every Tuesday, when her mother's copy of the *Journal of the American Medical Association* arrived in the mail, a twinge of guilt came with it. If not for Dominica, her mother would be a doctor. One night she brought this up with her mom, who just laughed.

"Why would I want to be a doctor when I can be a nurse? Doctors just give orders, like your dad," she added with a smile. "The nurses are the lucky ones. *We* do the caring."

"Then why do you get that journal?" asked Dominica with a nod at a copy.

Her mother grinned. "To have something to discuss with the doctors. They bore easily, you know."

Dominica didn't read *JAMA*, but COVID-19, she remembered, had appeared in the titles of several articles of a recent issue. Sure enough, in her parent's bedroom, Dominica spotted the journal on the bedstand on her mom's side of the bed.

April 7, 2020, page 1239: Characteristics of and Important Lessons From the Coronavirus Disease 2019 (COVID-19) Outbreak in China: Summary of a Report of 72,314 Cases From the Chinese Center for Disease Control and Prevention.

Dominica glanced through the article before focusing on a timeline on its final page.

COVID-19 outbreak 2019-2020

Dec. 8: First case

Onset of symptoms in the first known case of pneumonia with unknown etiology in Wuhan City, Hubei Province, China.

For Dominica, etiology was a new word. She guessed the meaning from the context but googled it on her phone to be sure.

Dec 31: Reported to WHO

China reports a cluster of cases of pneumonia with unknown etiology in Wuhan to WHO.

China:

27 cases

0 deaths

Jan 7: New Virus Identified

Chinese scientists identify the pathogen as a novel coronavirus.

Jan 30: WHO global alert

WHO declares a "public health emergency of international concern."

China:	Outside China:
7736 confirmed cases	82 confirmed cases
170 deaths	0 deaths

Dominica remembered her mother saying, months ago, about COVID, "This is going to be big." Was it back in January? Less clearly, she recalled her mother's irritation that the WHO had taken so long to declare an emergency. Had there been an earlier meeting of the WHO? Dominica googled it. Sure enough, on January 23.

She went back to the balcony and kept reading.

When asked about the President's directive, former White House communications chief Anthony Scaramucci (he was called the Mooch, her dad had said, for being "one of those money-for-nothing finance guys") wasn't surprised. "You can't underestimate this President," Scaramucci said. "Remember back in 2016 when no one expected him to win? Then, when his true colors became clear for everyone to see, after he'd sold out dozens of guys who'd worked for him, well, I said that it wouldn't be long until he sold out every American. But he's outdone himself. By not contributing to WHO, he's sold out the entire world."

The article was long and wide-ranging, and it took Dominica, paying close attention, twenty minutes to read. I.M. Wright, a professor at Dallas Theological Seminary, said, "We agree with the President. The WHO is part of a global cabal that now rules the entire planet. The Bible says that, like the destruction of the ancient city of Babylon, this global network must be destroyed before Jesus can return to earth."

Wright, a spokesman for Evangelicals for the President, continued, "You know, if you read the Bible, you'll find that God gave power to, let's just say, some unsavory characters. I mean, King David lusted almost as much as President Trump. The Lord works in mysterious ways. Our faith hasn't wavered. In this President we continue to trust."

Dominica set the paper down. How she wanted to discuss this with her mother! How she wanted her father well and home again!

Later that afternoon, she watched CNN, where a female journalist was asking people their opinions about the President's decision to defund the WHO. She caught up with John Q. Public in his office, where he worked as a CPA. "I don't know if I'm the right guy to ask," he said. "I'm basically a numbers guy, and I pretty much steer clear of politics. But it seems penny wise and pound foolish to me."

Next, she talked with Joe Sixpack, sitting on a lawn chair in front of his house, swigging a Miller Lite, facing into the sun. "You ever see the comedian who does this routine about a horse in a hospital?" he asked. "How the horse ain't supposed to be there, but because it is, and because you don't know what it's going to do next, and because the horse doesn't either, you can't stop watching? I think this is like that, only stranger, though for me, the strangeness is wearing thin. (Expletive deleted), I voted for him in 2016, but this time there ain't no way." Joe paused for a moment, took a swig from his can, and cracked a grin. "You remember four years ago, some people were saying he didn't really want to win? Just wanted publicity so he could make more money? Now, ya know, it's the only explanation that makes any sense. Trump wants to commit political suicide. He wants to (expletive deleted) lose." Joe let out a laugh from his big belly, broke out in a gap-toothed smile, and held up his beer can as if making a toast. "And you know what?" he asked. "I say go for it! (Expletive deleted) go for it!"

AS YOU DID IT FOR ONE
OF THE LEAST OF THESE
MY BROTHERS

April 16

At the dawn of 2020, the Life Care Center in Kirkland, Wash., cared for 120 residents. At its most recent state inspection, in April 2019, the nursing home received five stars, the federal government's highest rating, achieved by only 21 percent of U.S. long term care facilities. But during that survey, the Life Care Center was cited for failure to provide and implement an infection control policy. The deficiency wasn't considered serious, however, because if an issue were to occur, inspectors felt it would likely lead to merely "minimal harm or potential for harm." Now, 37 residents are dead.

I don't mean to denigrate the facility. I've seen their staff interviewed on television, and their devastation is palpable. And when you consider the circumstances of their outbreak, it's hard to cast blame.

The first two people in the United States to die from COVID, both on Feb. 26, had been residents of the center, though at the time no one knew that COVID had caused their deaths. Only later did epidemiologists determine the virus had been circulating in the area for several weeks.

In the waning days of February, residents started to spike fevers. They coughed, struggled to breathe. Some turned blue. You couldn't fault the staff for not considering COVID. Not then. Though the first U.S. COVID case was diagnosed on Jan. 20, it and all others since had been linked to travel from Wuhan. Tests weren't merely hard to come by, they were frowned upon, even prohibited. The CDC's directive was to screen patients for COVID only if they had specific symptoms—cough, fever, shortness of breath—*and* a travel history.

How often do we humans, creatures of habit, anticipate the unexpected? When the government tells us not to? (Testing in Wisconsin was no less of a challenge. In the first weeks of the pandemic, tests couldn't be ordered without permission from the state lab in Madison. After hours, you had to call and have somebody paged, which made it harder to detect community spread, or contagion in a nursing home. Such an early warning system, which would have been optimal, was precluded by a shortage of tests.)

There's a hierarchy in medicine. When a patient is admitted to a hospital or a long term care facility, nurses follow doctor's orders. They're even so named on the electronic health record. Physician order sets. Click-click-click-click-click.

Nurses are nice. They care, and do the caring, as noted yesterday. Doctors rely on them; in the hospital, they care for patients 24/7 while doctors attend them maybe 10 minutes a day. We collaborate, value their opinions, but when all's said and done, they do what we ask. Nurses, even the men, tend to be—dare I say?—obedient. So when nurses at Kirkland's Life Care Center were discouraged from suspecting COVID, in a sense they complied.

Most nursing homes, most of the time, don't have a physician on site. (For six years, I was a medical director at a local facility, where I saw patients and went to meetings on average two hours a week.) So don't blame the medical director at the Kirkland facility for not tumbling to COVID as the cause of its cluster of illnesses right from the start. Like the Chinese in Wuhan when the pandemic began, he was encountering an entirely unexpected—and for the Chinese, heretofore unknown—phenomenon.

Nursing homes are perfect contagion storms. According to the CDC, of 2,590 U.S. non-foodborne outbreaks of norovirus, the gastroenteritis common on cruise ships, from 2009-2012, 80 percent occurred in nursing homes.

In these places, special people work. Aides give baths, change soiled linens, and wipe butts, for less than $15/hour. To my mind, nurses and aides who choose careers in long term care facilities answer an almost religious calling. In a hospital, a nurse cares for five or six patients, while those in a home might have 30. Maybe there's not enough time to slip on the gloves and flimsy gowns that might not be available, or time enough even to wash your hands as often as you should. I've rounded in every area nursing home; adherence to infection control protocols, and PPE for staff, varies. But compared to hospitals, because they're under-resourced, nursing homes underperform.

Once COVID takes root in a long term care facility, it leaves a path of destruction in its wake. Nursing homes are filled with elderly and debilitated patients burdened with an abundance of chronic disease, each of which are risk factors for poor COVID outcomes. Like cholera in healthy people, COVID can kill the infirm in mere hours.

New York City recently revised upwards its COVID death toll by 3,800, many of whom died in nursing homes before a definitive diagnosis could be made. In NYC, most nursing home patients presumed to have succumbed to the virus died before a test could be administered.

At Fairview Rehab and Nursing Home in Queens, a nurse said the facility, in recent weeks, had run out of room to store bodies. "We know it's because of the virus because it's people who've been here for years, who suddenly can't breathe. They die very quickly."

Ninety percent of New Jersey's nursing homes have had a documented COVID case. At the state's veterans' home, 27 patients have died, and almost half of the survivors are either COVID positive or awaiting confirmation of the same. National Guard medics have been brought in to replace sick staff.

In Elizabeth, population 130,000, the virus is known to have killed 65 residents in three separate facilities.

In Andover, also in New Jersey, police acted on an anonymous tip and discovered seventeen bodies in a small morgue intended for four or less. These 17 deaths were among 68 recently at Andover's rehab center, 26 of them confirmed from COVID. Of the surviving patients, 76 are COVID positive, in addition to 41 staff. (The care center is licensed for 700 beds, the largest in the state.)

At the Symphony of Joliet, an assisted living facility in that Chicago suburb, COVID has killed 22 residents.

Nearly half of the deaths attributed to the virus in Massachusetts have been in nursing homes.

As of two days ago, the federal government counted 3,600 deaths across the country in nursing homes or assisted living facilities, up from several hundred just days before.

According to David Grabowski, a professor of health policy at Harvard, the figure is actually "much higher," in part because of the dearth of testing cited above. In addition, Grabowski says, there's no federal mechanism to track deaths in care facilities. While "some states have done a great job in tracking these (COVID) cases and these deaths, other states are doing nothing," he says.

For the states that track causes of death, record keepers depend on what doctors write on death certificates. If it doesn't say "pneumonia from COVID," or "pneumonia from suspected COVID," it doesn't count.

We should have seen this coming. The Life Care Center of Kirkland, Wash. was ground zero for COVID in the United States. But our hustle-bustle American life, though good at generating wealth, fares poorly at planning ahead. And in America, taking care of our most vulnerable has never been a high priority.

A GOOD MASK IS
HARD TO FIND

April 17

Six weeks ago, I was torn. For several days I struggled with what I should do. Finally, I made up my mind.

On March 6, I googled N95 masks. Most of the suppliers were out of stock, but some guy with an American name—Bob, maybe; I don't remember what he called himself or his "business"—had a 10 pack for sale.

So I took out my credit card and paid for the masks: $134.98. Thirteen and a half bucks a mask, the best price I could find. (I was told by someone in my employer's supply chain, through whom I was trying to procure N95s for our free clinic, that in normal times the masks sold for less than a dollar each.)

I know, I know, I shouldn't have. The masks are needed by frontline providers, the doctors and nurses caring for patients with COVID. But wasn't I a doctor? And my employer had made a big deal about not having enough N95s; we had to conserve them; they were reserved for "aerosol-generating procedures" such as nebulizer treatments on patients with a definite COVID diagnosis; mere breathing or talking isn't considered an AGP, despite a fair amount of evidence that it is. If you wore an N95 when management didn't deem it appropriate, you could be cited—management had already done so, they emphasized—for "failure to work," prelude, possibly, to being terminated.

Compliance, you know. If Dr. S. is wearing an N95, Nurse N. will want to, too, and the stockpile will dwindle until there really aren't enough.

But I wasn't merely thinking of myself, though it crossed my mind to abscond with maybe half of the masks, should I get the chance to serve in New York or New Jersey, a request formally made to my employer and as formally denied. I'm required to "work" from home, phoning a few patients, paid for eight hours but engaged perhaps two, and they need me to prepare for a local surge that isn't coming. Why do some have so little and others so much?

My mother turned 90 this week, my father will be 90 soon—they started dating at fourteen and were married at 21. My-ex wife is a nurse in Lexington, Ken.; my oldest son lives with her and works as a nurse's aide; my wife's mother is elderly and lives alone. Didn't they need masks, too?

The good physician, said H.L. Mencken, confers absolution without demanding redemption. (Mencken, who liked his cocktails, must have had a *very* good physician.)

Won't you be, won't you be…my physician?

I digress, as my long-suffering friends will attest.

Time passed. A good two weeks. I almost forgot I'd ordered the masks. (In truth, I figured I'd been scammed.) Served me right! And why keep reminding myself of my stupidity, which it was best to forget.

But then, an email informed me my items had shipped! Bob, or whoever he was, *wasn't* a scoundrel—true, he'd marked up my masks beaucoup—because the N95s weren't merely on their way to me but on their way from afar! Across the vast Pacific, from China. The city of Fuzhou, in Fujian Province, to be exact. My estimation of Bob leapt into the stratosphere. Dude was resourceful.

Bob, my email said, "might" have tracking information for my order, but it wasn't possible to get in touch with him.

No need. I had faith.

That was a month ago. Over the ensuing two weeks, I drifted from eager anticipation to—more or less—stoic resignation. My masks weren't coming. The logistics of transport from China had to be complicated, and my package would have had many opportunities to get lost in the mail. And I thought that, just maybe, my marked-up masks had become a pawn, albeit teeny-tiny, in a geopolitical chess match. Perhaps, in retaliation for POTUS's trade war, the Chinese were holding onto them—a megalomaniacal fantasy that fortunately for me and my patients was short-lived.

(A week ago, the *New York Times* reported Chinese officials had begun inspecting every shipment of N95s for quality issues prior to export, a policy predicted to delay shipment of this critical gear to hospitals across the globe. The new regs came after European complaints that some Chinese N95s weren't medical grade. There'd been rumors—see my unmoored musings above—that political considerations had prevented the masks from being shipped, but the buzz wasn't true. From March 1 through April 4, according to the *Times*, China exported 3.86 billion masks.)

Be all of this as it may, I'd given up on getting my greedy hands on any masks, of Chinese or whatever provenance. And it wasn't as if there was nothing else to think about. The world was turning topsy-turvy, and I had to keep up!

So I was surprised when, earlier this week, a package came in the mail. Surprised and titillated, even. A package for me? What could it be? I couldn't remember ordering anything. That it could contain my N95s didn't occur.

The package was soft and squishy to the touch—clearly not a book from Amazon, basically the only non-letter mail I ever get. (After hearing the novelist Julia Glass discuss her loathing of Amazon, for ripping off authors, I'd tried Barnes and Noble. But on my second B&N order, I received an explicit graphic novel instead of the literary one I *swear* I'd ordered, and I switched back. Say what you will about Amazon, they're great at logistics.)

My wife shared my excitement as I beamed at the package held out in my hands. Oh, boy!

I tore into it and found…a sports bra, pretty and powder blue.

Oh, shit! was my first thought. A former girlfriend's final act of spite. (I don't know why this popped into my head, but it did.) But not only could I not recall the bra, it appeared brand new. And the return address on the package, when I put on my glasses and peered close, was Fuzhou, Fujian, China.

I suppose I could file a complaint with American Express, or the Bureau of Consumer Protection, but I think I'll keep it.

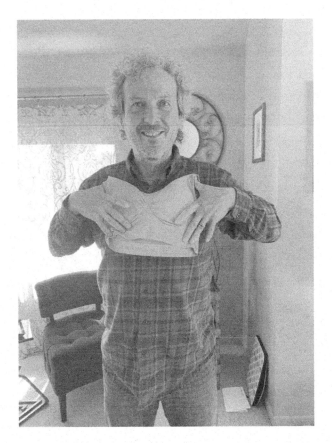

The author with his Chinese sports bra

PANDEMIC PSYCHOLOGY

April 18

On Feb. 27, two days before the CDC reported the first American death from COVID, I sat in a board meeting of the local YMCA, of which I'm a director. A few months earlier, under the guidance of our executive director, Theresa Hillis, the board made the heartbreaking decision to drop out of a project to build a joint facility with Mayo and UW-Eau Claire. We couldn't come up with the cash for our part of the deal.

On that late February day, prelude to constructing a new "Y," or remodeling our current facility, Theresa outlined the necessary steps for a successful capital campaign. She pointed out several possible challenges: obtaining broad community buy-in, one or two major donors, ten or twelve others who could pony up half a million or more, and several dozen citizens whose "philanthropic urge"—in the apt words of Dick Cable, a longtime community benefactor—might be channeled into a gift of perhaps 50k. We needed support for the building site. Donors had to be convinced they'd get their money's worth. None of these preconditions were assured. Were there other potential obstacles, Theresa asked?

I raised my hand. (Actually, I'm afraid I didn't. In meetings, I tend to just open my big mouth if I've got something to say.)

"Well," I said, "if this virus thing gets going, all bets are off."

I mentioned the work of Mark Lipsitch, the Harvard epidemiologist who earlier in the month had predicted a pandemic in which 40 to 70 percent of the world's population would be infected. In late February, the WHO quoted a mortality rate of 3.4 percent—deaths divided by documented cases. (Now, using the same math, the death rate is exactly double, but since the true denominator, because of uncounted cases, is likely higher by at least a factor of ten, the actual mortality rate is probably lower by that same order of magnitude.)

I tossed out some scary and hastily calculated numbers—which I got wrong and revised downward minutes later—of how many Americans might die.

"We're not ready for that," I said.

Across the room from me, local health department director and fellow board member Lieske Giese nodded her head.

"Even if the figures are only 10 percent of what I quoted," I continued, "the psychological consequences will be profound. Not only will people pull away, withdraw from the world, they'll hide within themselves. Psychological retrenchment. They won't spend money, and they won't want to give it, either."

Needless to say, our capital campaign, the campaign for the local public library, and countless similar campaigns across the globe have been put on hold.

No doubt it would be difficult to raise money for a building project when the campaign's object had closed its doors, and a plunging stock market—though not plunging too much; more on this later—has made benefactors feel less wealthy and not as willing to give.

Difficult, but not impossible. But there's a sense that capital campaigns would be uphill slogs, so leaders are quitting before they begin.

Yesterday afternoon, on the bike trail in downtown Eau Claire, I walked upstream beside the Chippewa. The sun was bright, but a chill breeze blew off the river. In front of me, a woman marched ahead. When someone passed her the other way, she moved off the trail and onto the grass, always six feet apart.

We were walking into the wind, and she didn't hear me approach. I caught up to her beneath the Lake Street Bridge, keeping myself as far away as was possible.

"Hi," I said, maintaining my pace.

She froze, turned to me with fear in her eyes, and said nothing. I kept moving.

I don't mean to be critical. Each of us has a unique risk tolerance, and we doctor types, to keep the virus at bay, don't mind if people are afraid of the virus, just a bit. Whomever she sees, her dread will help keep them safe.

This avoidance mindset isn't only physical. It can turn into an inability to engage, and not wanting to. Sheltering at home may abet self-absorption, psychological cloistering mimicking the physical, as if everyone is growing old and frail all at once.

These last two weeks, I've seen few patients. My workday consists of answering computer queries and making phone calls. We've switched most of our encounters from face-to-face to phone or video.

Eighty percent of my patients are over 65. Many haven't been out of their homes in weeks. Some tell me their children forbid them to. At the clinic, our numbers are down, and not just a little. Our appointment fill rates have dropped by a third. We're reaching out to patients, but they're declining our invitations.

Some of my colleagues consider this strange. But if you consider pandemic psychology, a hunker-down mentality, it makes sense. Our local health care leaders warn of another surge in the coming weeks, when patients with unmet needs will want to be seen.

Like the predicted surge into the hospital, I don't think it will materialize. In addition to psychological retrenchment, we've turned the clinic (barricaded pharmacy, entrance festooned with warning signs) into a frightening place. It may take time for patients to return; health care demand may be more elastic than some administrators think. Perhaps we won't ever be as popular as we once were.

A 91-year-old man I spoke with yesterday stood out from his hibernating peers; he's exceptional in general. Each Sunday, he's one of four in church along with a pastor, an organist, and a soloist. In Wisconsin, when the churches are allowed to open again on May 31, don't expect the pews to be filled.

The city of Wuhan, China, has reopened. Its 11 million people are free to dine out. But they're not. For culinary entrepreneur Xiong Fei, instead of relief, the end of the lockdown has brought a new set of challenges.

"People in the past dined out with their colleagues in their lunch hour," he said. "Now they're all getting lunch boxes. They're more likely to cook at home than go out." Xiong fears the changes in behavior may be permanent.

Since the stock market close on Monday, March 16, the S&P 500 is up more than 20 percent. During this time, the American economy has shed 22 million jobs. One in seven Americans is newly out of work. Former Fed Chief Janet Yellen says that "unemployment may go to depression levels." (It peaked at 25% in 1933.) Never has the disconnect between Wall Street and Main Street been as stark.

Analysts searching for an explanation have landed on the expectation of a "V"-shaped recovery. Yes, they say, there will be economic pain, but the suffering will be short-lived.

In the U.S., 70 percent of GDP is driven by consumer spending, a figure high by historical standards. In Japan, the number is 55 percent, in Germany, 52 percent, in China just 39 percent.

Investors think that in a few months people will be back at work, making money, and spending it like never before.

On this hypothesis, I wouldn't bet my life savings.

SMITHFIELD: CRADLE OF CRUELTY

April 19

On July 16, 1534, Anne Askew—given recent renown in Hilary Mantel's Booker Prize-winning *Wolf Hall*—was burned at the stake. A great stage was built at Smithfield, just outside of London's gates, to allow Chancellor Wriothesley, other members of the Privy Council, and assorted city dignitaries to watch the burning in comfort. Anne, broken by the rack and unable to stand, was chained to the stake in a sitting position.

The Archdeacon of Nottingham witnessed the execution and described an angelic Anne smiling throughout her torment. At the moment of her death, he insisted there was a "pleasant cracking from heaven." Whether this was the sound of the flames, summer lightning or a figment of the Archbishop's imagination couldn't be discerned, nor could, given the gruesome manner of her death, the precise second when her heart ceased to beat.

Why was Anne murdered? She refused to recant her Protestant beliefs.

Smithfield, Va.—located on the banks of the believe-it-or-not Pagan River and not far from Jamestown—was colonized in 1634. Years earlier, John Smith—*that* John Smith—first explored the area. Smith himself was from Lincolnshire, 100 miles north of London. Though he'd have known of his nation's Smithfield, I suspect he gave *his* name to the Virginia settlement;

anyone who kills and beheads three Ottomans in separate duels has an ego. But the provenance of the city's name isn't known with certainty.

Founded in 1936 as the Smithfield Packing Company, in Smithfield, Va., Smithfield Foods is the largest pork producer in the world. In addition to owning over 500 U.S. farms, Smithfield contracts with an additional 2,000 independent farms to grow pigs.

Each day at the Smithfield plant in Sioux Falls, S.D., 3,700 workers process 19,500 slaughtered hogs. On the line, workers stand inches apart. The vast majority are immigrants—80 different languages swarm the factory's air—doing work that native-born Americans won't deign to do. Most hail from Nepal or Latin America (20 years ago, while trekking in the Himalaya, I watched in awe as 120-pound, bare-foot porters carried 90-pound loads secured by tump lines across their foreheads over rocky trails, the most extraordinary feat of physical and mental stamina I've ever seen) though the website of the Sioux Falls cultural center also has COVID info in Arabic, Bosnian, Amharic (a Semitic offshoot, and the official language of Ethiopia), Somali, French, Croatian, Kunama (between Eritrea and Ethiopia), Russian, and Swahili.

Ahmed first saw Neela on the Smithfield floor during one of their shifts. He liked her skin, she liked his laugh. He asked around about her and found she was from the same village in Ethiopia.

"Wow, I'm so excited," Ahmed said. "In my breaktime, I keep searching where she work. Right away, I stop by her line. I say, 'Hey, what's up?' I tell her she's beautiful."

He took her to a trendy restaurant. They took a week-long vacation in Wisconsin Dells. They fell in love and were married.

Neela, who no longer works on the line, is eight months pregnant. Recently, she started having trouble walking. Ahmed needs to help her; they can't social distance. Two of his friends at the plant have tested COVID positive. Ahmed has started showing symptoms of the virus himself.

Rosa is a grad student who returned to Sioux Falls after her college closed. Though she doesn't work at the plant, her parents, who don't speak English, do. On March 25, Rosa sat down at her laptop, logged into a fake Facebook account, and typed a message to Argus911, the FB-tip line for the *Argus Leader*, the local newspaper. "Can you please look into Smithfield? They do have a positive (COVID) case and are planning to stay open."

The paper confirmed her story and published it the next day. Smithfield responded that the employee in question was in a 14-day quarantine, and his work area and other common spaces had been "thoroughly sanitized."

A week earlier, Smithfield CEO Kenneth Sullivan said, "Food is an essential part of all our lives, and our more than 40,000 U.S. team members, thousands of American family farmers and our many other supply chain partners are a crucial part of our nation's response to COVID-19. We are taking the utmost precautions to ensure the health and well-being of our employees and consumers."

Sullivan was lying. According to Taneeza Islam, an immigration attorney in Sioux Falls who has worked with Smithfield employees, "there was no social distancing occurring on the lines from at least before March 26 to when some measures like taking temperatures outside of the plant before employees had to come in took place on Monday, April 6. So for that period of time, we know that mitigation efforts were not taking place."

Even the temperature checks could be circumvented by employees choosing to enter through a side door. On April 9, the day after the South Dakota State Health Department confirmed 80 cases at the plant, Smithfield announced the factory would close for deep cleaning over the three-day Easter weekend. Company-dispensed PPE consisted of beard nets, worthless against a virus whose diameter is less than a micron.

According to the BBC, the plant stayed open Easter weekend, running at close to two-thirds capacity. On April 11, Sioux Falls Mayor Paul Tenhaken and South Dakota Governor Kristi Noem, both Republicans, sent a joint letter to Smithfield calling for a 14-day "pause" in operations. The company said it would comply, but didn't until April 15, when the virus had already infected 644 Smithfield employees or contacts. During the two-week closure, workers would be paid and also offered a "responsibility bonus" of $500 for returning to work after the pause.

Agriculture Secretary Sonny Perdue responded to Smithfield's announcement by praising "the true commitment and patriotism our food supply chain workers have shown during this time and the work they continue to do day in and day out."

Rosa's parents were both scheduled to work April 14, the final day before the shutdown. But three days earlier, her mother started to cough. She insisted it was nothing, but Rosa convinced her to get a COVID test.

"If I were to have COVID," said her mother through Rosa, "I clearly would have gotten it at the factory. This week I have worked on three different floors. I've eaten in two different cafeterias. I've been walking through the whole place."

On April 14, Rosa's parents woke at four a.m. per usual and called Smithfield to say they couldn't work until they'd received her mother's results. Later that afternoon, they got the call: positive.

It's hard not to equate Smithfield's offer of a $500 "responsibility bonus" with the value of an immigrant's life. Few employees have talked to the media; whether Smithfield has prohibited them to or they're scared isn't clear; the BBC changed the names in the above narrative to prevent reprisals against the women and men.

Every immigrant, even a visa holder, could be considered a public charge, at risk for deportation, if she quits and files for unemployment, thanks to a 2019 rule by the Trump Administration preventing her from obtaining permanent citizenship. In addition, the recent Coronavirus Aid, Relief, and Economic Security (CARES) Act excludes anyone living in a family with an undocumented immigrant.

Smithfield employees have no choice. They need to work and risk exposure to the virus in order to put the pork they process on their kitchen tables. Meat processing workers have joined communities of color and nursing home residents in extreme vulnerability to COVID's ravages.

It's nothing new. Marginalized people always suffer the most.

WARRIORS, IN THE ARMY OR IN HOSPITALS, NEED PROTECTION

April 20

Mike Gulick didn't want to contract COVID. Because he has diabetes, he's at higher risk for serious disease. Nor did he want to give it to his wife or two-year-old daughter. Each day after work, he'd stop at a hotel to shower before driving home. Until a few days ago, Gulick worked as a nurse at Providence St. John's Health Center in Santa Monica.

Angela Gatdula, another St. John's nurse, had asked hospital managers why doctors were wearing N95 masks while nurses couldn't. She was told that, according to the CDC, surgical masks were sufficient. So, when she took care of patients with COVID, that's what she wore. Then she came down with a dry cough and severe body aches.

"When I got the phone call that I was positive," she said, "I got really scared." She's recovering at home and plans to return to work soon. "The next nurse that gets this might not be lucky. They might require hospitalization. They might die."

The day after Gulick found out about Gatdula, doctors rounding on his floor wondered why he wasn't wearing an N95. Nurses should have better protection, they said. For Gulick, it flipped a switch. He and nine nurse colleagues told their supervisor they wouldn't work without N95 masks when caring for patients with COVID.

"I went into nursing with a passion for helping those who are most vulnerable and being an advocate for those who couldn't have a voice for themselves, but not under the condition we're currently under," he said.

One at a time, Gulick and his colleagues were called into a meeting with hospital administrators, who read the same script to each nurse. Management told them their refusal to treat patients constituted negligence and abandonment. If they continued to refuse, the administrators said, the nurses would be reported to the California Board of Registered Nursing, a threat they carried out. They asked each nurse to treat patients three successive times. When the nurses demurred, they were suspended and asked to leave the building.

"We all said to them, no, we're not refusing the assignment, we're refusing to take care of these patients without the minimal protection of an N95 mask," Gulick said. "And they said, we cannot provide that to you."

Across the nation, at least 9,200 health care workers (HCWs) have been sickened by the virus. In the initial weeks of Europe's epidemic, 14 percent of Spain's cases were HCWs, while the figure in Italy was one in 10.

Gulick and his colleagues are among hundreds across the country who've publicly complained about inadequate protection while caring for patients with COVID. I say *publicly* complained, because at many institutions, including mine, employees are forbidden to talk to the media. A complaint from Oregon alleged nurses were told "wearing an N95 mask will result in disciplinary action."

My employer appears to agree with the administrators of this Oregon facility. Staff wearing N95s for other than institution-approved indications, which don't include routine care to patients with documented COVID infection, could be cited for "failure to work," prelude to possible termination. Recently, our Wisconsin supply chain manager stated we had an inventory of 5 million N95 masks. There are only two inpatients with COVID in our five northwest Wisconsin hospitals combined, both at my place of work. In Eau

Claire County, there's been just one new COVID case in the last two weeks. No surge is soon forthcoming; for the coming weeks, five million masks will be more than enough.

Across the U.S., exasperated HCWs have complained to OSHA, while others have taken to the streets. Nurses in New York, Massachusetts, Michigan, Illinois, California, and Pennsylvania have staged protests outside of their hospitals, and they've posted on social media #PPEoverProfit.

The fallback for hospital administrators is that they're providing PPE according to CDC guidelines. But from the start, these guidelines have plenty of gray. Facing a worldwide shortage of N95s, the CDC said last month that surgical masks could be used instead. If surgical masks aren't available, HCPs can try bandannas.

Now the CDC says N95s are "preferred" when caring for patients with COVID. If we had enough N95s, if POTUS used the Defense Production Act to make billions, this would be a non-issue. But POTUS won't lead.

We've been told that COVID is mostly transmitted by respiratory droplets, coughed or sneezed by patients (though sneezing isn't common with COVID) and falling to the ground within a six-foot radius. But this is simplistic, says increasing evidence.

After the COVID outbreak on the aircraft carrier U.S.S. Roosevelt, each sailor on the ship got a test. 60 percent of infected servicemen had no symptoms. Thousands of police and first responders in the urban northeast have taken sick. Were most of them coughed upon?

I don't think so. In my opinion, they were *breathed* upon.

We know that COVID is at least three times more contagious than the flu. Why is it more transmissible? At least part of the reason, in my view, is that the virus can be transmitted by aerosol. Again in my opinion, we've made people too paranoid about contact with contaminated surfaces—a mode not known to have caused a single case of COVID, even though proving something never happens is exceedingly hard—and not anxious enough about inhaling the virus. If you're a nurse taking care of a patient infected with COVID, an N95 is your safest choice.

The right PPE for the right occasion, my employer says. Starting today, every patient, nurse, and provider will wear a surgical mask. This is great! My mask protects my patients, while theirs protects me. If either is negligent, the other's at risk. The strategy should be expanded to grocery and convenience stores and every retail outlet in the land. All for one and one for all. If they can do it in Singapore and South Korea, we can too!

But our supreme leader won't help. He's not capable. Instead of a United States of America, a Divided States of America is what he seeks.

BEWARE OF HOSPITALS!

April 21

A friend of mine was worried about his dad, a longtime patient. The man is in his 80s and lives with his wife in a ranch-style home. Last Sunday, I made a house call.

Their home faces south. The sky was a brilliant blue, and the late morning sun, bathing their yard in light, took the chill out of the air. Their grass was greener than any I'd seen this year.

My friend, wearing a mask, sat on the deck in front of the house. He stood to greet me as his mother walked outside, her arms spread wide.

"Oh, Steve," she said. "How I'd like to hug you!"

For now, hugs are a thing of the past.

I'd met my friend in first grade. After school, I used to hang at his house, shooting baskets in the driveway, while his mother made chocolate chip cookies that we gorged on when we were done. Through high school, we kept shooting hoops. More truthfully, I sat at the end of the bench and watched him drain swishes from the top of the key.

His father had moved the family north from Iowa to take an entry-level position at a large Eau Claire institution. When he became my patient 20-plus years ago, he'd recently retired as its CEO. At the clinic, whenever I walked into an exam room to see him, he'd rise from his chair and look into my eyes with his bright blues.

"Dr. Weiss," he'd say, as he shook my hand.

To be honest, though not his intent (he's humble as a servant and always polite) it was a bit intimidating. His calm self-assurance made me less confident, because I don't move through the world with his seeming ease. Think Colin Powell, only mellower. In the 40-plus years my dad was a dentist, my friend's dad was one of two patients who'd fallen asleep while my father worked on him.

In the living room, my patient sat on the couch, a bathrobe over his bare chest, making it easier for me to examine him. I sat in an adjacent chair, his wife heated coffee in the kitchen, and my friend sat outside on the deck, the sliding door to the living room open so he could hear what we said.

My patient's complaints, in medical vernacular, were non-specific, not pointing to a particular cause. Weakness, weight loss, swollen feet. His chronic cough hadn't changed. I examined him, recommended blood tests and x-rays. They could be done, I thought, in the next day or two.

My patient took in this counsel in his typical thoughtful manner before he asked, "Are you worried about the coronavirus?"

"No," I replied, less thoughtfully. "You don't really have symptoms. And you haven't been anywhere to catch it."

He hadn't been out of his house in a month. My friend bought groceries for his parents, handed them to his mother across the threshold, refused to venture into the house. From the deck, my friend said, "I don't think he's worried that he *has* the coronavirus. I think he's worried about getting it at the hospital."

One glance at my patient confirmed my friend's hunch. He'd be given a mask at the hospital, I reassured him, where everyone else would wear one too. Universal masking, I explained, would keep him safe.

He nodded.

Logistics were discussed, we bid our farewells, and I walked out. As my friend closed the sliding door, he turned to his mother and said, "Be sure to wipe the door handle clean."

My patient is an intelligent man. If *he* was worried about going to a clinic, who isn't?

Not just those needing tests or due for routine checkups, it turns out. At NYC's Mt. Sinai hospital, cardiac surgeon John Puskas wonders where all the heart patients have gone. Even patients with crushing chest pain weren't calling 911. A recent report in the *Journal of the American College of Cardiology* from nine cardiac cath labs across the country found a 38 percent drop in patients being treated for the most severe type of myocardial infarction (MI), medicalese for heart attack. Wouldn't the stress of a pandemic cause more MIs? To my mind, possible changes in diet or exercise can't explain the significant drop. Instead patients seem to prefer suffering and maybe dying from an MI to going to a hospital they consider more dangerous.

Evert Eriksson, the trauma medical director at the Medical University of South Carolina (MUSC), describes a man in his 20s who tried to ignore the growing pain in his abdomen, toughing it out at home, loading up on painkillers. When the patient finally showed up at the hospital, 10 days after he should have, his burst appendix had caused a large abscess that was eating into his abdominal muscles.

"What we're seeing is late presentation," Eriksson said. "I would say 70 percent of the appendicitis on my service right now are late presentations. What happens when you present late with appendicitis is we can't operate on you safely. We have five COVID patients in the hospital right now, and we have five appendicitis cases with complications from waiting too long to seek care."

MUSC's stroke center averages 550 calls a month from referring ERs. In the first half of April, the number is under a hundred. At the University of Miami-Jackson Stroke Center, the census in March was down 30 percent from the month before.

A Gallup poll taken March 28 to April 2 asked people how concerned they'd be about exposure to COVID if they needed "medical treatment right now" at a clinic or hospital. 86 percent of people with heart disease said they'd be moderately or very concerned. For high blood pressure, the figure was 83 percent.

As an outpatient internal medicine doc, probably 80 percent of my practice is wellness checks and what we term chronic disease management, surveillance of, for instance, diabetes, hypertension, and heart disease. If patients don't want to go to the hospital for emergencies, they won't come to the clinic for routine care. My employer wants our practice up and running at 100 percent of usual utilization by June 1, which seems ambitious. In a full morning today at the office, I saw one patient and called one more. The words of Dr. Birx warning people to be wary of contaminated surfaces (reinforced by the likes of Dr. Oz), reports of nurses sickened by the virus, and the images of bodies piling up outside of a Queens hospital, may have been seared into patients' brains.

It's not only the fear factor. Part of the explanation is the psychological retrenchment discussed before, withdrawing into oneself. Not only are people staying home, the new routine is becoming more comfortable. Business travel is down dramatically, vacations have been postponed, and consumers aren't buying new houses or cars. It's as if, across the country, collective desire has taken a hit.

It's a scary proposition for a nation where consumer spending accounts for 70 percent of the economy, a figure that both leads the world and is high by U.S. historical standards.

Decreased desire may partly explain why oil prices have plummeted. And rather than surging 700-plus points because of hopeful information from uncontrolled trials about the anti-viral drug Remdesivir and the announcement of a trio of steps taken by POTUS to reopen the economy, a process he can't control, the stock market is responding to actual data.

Nizar Tarhuni is director of research and analysis for Pitchbook, a newsletter tracking private equity.

"Everyone who's in these (oil futures) contracts who thought oil would rebound by now, they're just dumping everything," Tarhuni said. "This structural scenario of the oil industry nowadays, I've never seen anything worse."

A possible silver lining? Mr. Tarhuni is just 28.

THE PERILS AND ALLURE
OF INSULARITY

April 22

Psychological retrenchment isn't limited to individuals. Vacation destinations have told tourists to stay away. A 30-second clip from the East Coast features an overhead panorama of an empty beach.

"Ocean City, Maryland, isn't the same without you. But rest assured, when it's finally time to come out again, we'll be here waiting. The lifeguards and the tram drivers. The folks making French fries and funnel cakes. The guys running ski ball and mini golf. The waiters and the waitresses. The hotel clerks and the T-shirt vendors. We're all excited to see you. But until then, stay healthy."

In essence, the ad tells people to stay away. (The activities described served that purpose for me.) Jessica Waters, Ocean City's tourism director, says, "You know, really, we don't have the resources here to handle a large amount of sick people."

Hayward, Wis., is home to the American Birkebeiner, the largest cross-country ski race in North America, thousands of lycra-clad Nordic enthusiasts taking the annual 50-kilometer trek. The Hayward area is awash in clear lakes and hilly woodlands laced with trails for skiing, snowshoeing, and mountain biking. It's a mecca for silent sports fans and fishermen. Each weekend hundreds commute to area cabins.

With a population of 2,300, Hayward is the largest community in Sawyer County, which in the last two weeks reported its first two COVID cases. Both were "community spread," the infectious contacts for them unknown. A month ago, before the pair was diagnosed, the Hayward Area Chamber of Commerce released a directive from Sawyer County Health and Human Services:

"Due to high community transmission in certain areas of the State, the Sawyer County Public Health Officer recommends that you stay in your permanent home and not travel to your seasonal or second home in Sawyer County. Due to the very limited health care infrastructure, please do not visit us now."

By that logic, those of us with cabins in the vicinity ought to stay away for at least the next year and a half.

This insular shift is most marked at the level of nation-states. Let's start with POTUS, exemplar extraordinaire. Earlier he closed the border with Mexico, announcing that undocumented workers would be turned back. Now, on green cards, he's turned the semaphore red. Want to bring your brains and brawn and desire for a better life to the United States? We don't want you! Stay away! Business and agriculture erupted in protest, and POTUS backed off a wee bit. Or perhaps his second thoughts were more self-centered. Who would pick his fruit? (Not that fruit is a staple of his diet.) Slaughter his hogs? Process his bacon? How could POTUS pig out?

"Well, I don't necessarily agree with it," said Stephen Colbert of his plan, "but it probably is the safest thing for immigrants. Because right now, America is basically a petri dish on the floor of a bus station men's room."

"We are fighting a two-front war," says Hungarian Prime Minister Viktor Orban. "One front is called migration and the other one belongs to the coronavirus. There is a logical connection between the two as both spread with movement."

In 1985, seven European nations created the Schengen Area (the agreement was signed in Schengen, Luxembourg), which abolished internal borders and visa requirements, marking the inception of the now 26-nation European Union. On March 17, the EU closed its borders, and many member countries, before or since, have followed suit. Belgium sealed itself off more than a month ago. Now, at 540 deaths per million inhabitants, Belgium has the highest COVID mortality rate in the world. The WHO that POTUS defunded opposes travel restrictions in pandemics for one basic reason. They don't work.

Not only have nation-states retrenched, authoritarian leaders like Orban, perhaps mindful of the Chinese proverb, have opportunistically used the COVID crisis to enhance their power. On March 30, Hungary's parliament voted by a two-thirds majority to let him rule by decree. No new elections may be held, certain laws need not be enforced, and anyone publicizing "untrue or distorted facts" faces a prison term.

In Israel Benjamin Netanyahu is up to similar tricks. Facing trial for corruption, he shut down the judiciary. His Likud Party closed Parliament rather than allow a vote on his successor, who in all likelihood would have come from the Blue and White Alliance, narrow winners of the election on March 2. If his power play bothers Israelis, they can't take to the streets. As in most countries, new regulations prevent public gatherings.

China has expelled U.S. journalists. According to Human Rights Watch, the Chinese have detained domestic reporters who've tried to travel to Wuhan. Thailand, Cambodia, Bangladesh, Venezuela, and Turkey have followed China's lead, arresting journalists, opposition activists, health care workers, anyone daring to criticize the COVID response of their governments.

Power is in love with itself. Never is the narcissism more apparent than in an emergency, real or imagined, when power is unleashed to accumulate more. Corporations aren't immune to this dynamic, where power arrogates to the (typically) men at the top.

For the last several weeks, my organization has presented twice weekly virtual town hall meetings, valuable forums for information-sharing and addressing employees' concerns. Questions are posed on Slido, where you can see other queries and vote on those you'd like answered. Yesterday, someone wrote, "The CDC now says N95 masks are preferred for routine care of COVID positive patients. There won't be a surge. Why doesn't Mayo change its policy?"

It was a question in which I had an interest. The underlying logic seemed sound, and I gave it an online thumbs-up. In Wisconsin, we'd been social distancing for more than a month, there'd been only one new COVID case in our county in a fortnight, we had just one COVID patient in our hospital, and the manager of our supply chain reassured us that we had an abundance of N95s.

The man who answered the anonymous question is a fine human being. "First of all," he said. "I need to make a correction. There won't be a surge is far too certain a statement. And the reason why we're not changing our policy," he added, pique slipping into his tone, "is because of what I just said. Whether or not we have a surge depends on you. Keep doing a great job by practicing social distancing."

That was the end of the dialogue. In a non-COVID environment, I can imagine the questioner, in the 250-seat auditorium where such forums are held, following up: "In Wisconsin, we'll have five more weeks of mandated social distancing. Do you have data, maybe from modeling, to suggest there's still a risk of a surge?"

"How many N95s are on hand?"

"Out of an abundance of caution, wouldn't it make sense to allow nurses caring for our single COVID patient to use his or her N95?"

But the virtual format precluded the possibility.

The scenario above more widely applies. Great companies find ways to not only welcome but encourage varied viewpoints. COVID, by decreasing face-to-face meetings, may impede corporate success.

In response to the pandemic, turning inward—nations, communities, corporations, and individuals—has become the norm. Does it have to be this way? Eventually, the pandemic will touch everyone in the world. Instead of retrenching, shouldn't we be reaching out? Building bridges? Forging new connections? Binding more tightly our existing ties? Supporting the health organization that spans the globe?

John Donne said it best.

No man is an island,

Entire of itself.

Each is a piece of the continent,

A part of the main.

If a clod be washed away by the sea,

Europe is the less.

As well as if a promontory were.

As well as if a manor of thine own

Or of thine's friend were.

Each man's death diminishes me,

For I am involved in mankind.

Therefore, send not to know

For whom the bell tolls,

It tolls for thee.

THE WAR NOT WAGED

April 23

Harvey Fineberg received his M.D. and Ph.D. from Harvard, where he's had a long and distinguished career. A former Dean of the Harvard School of Public Health and President of the Institute of Medicine, Dr. Fineberg is the chair of the Standing Committee on Emerging Infectious Diseases and 21st Century Threats. On NPR recently, he was asked about the necessary conditions to reopen the economy. I've edited his response for length and clarity.

"These conditions," he said, "are not simply conditions that you wait for. They're conditions that you help create. The first fundamental condition is doing adequate testing in order to do two things—detect anyone who's infected and, secondly, survey the community to detect any escalation in cases. Number two, every community that plans to relax social distancing needs to be able to contain any escalation and, in addition, treat newly ill patients. This capacity to contain depends on the ability to trace anyone who is newly infected."

Former CDC director Tom Friedan has said we need 300,000 workers for this purpose, and current CDC director Robert Redfield has suggested that census workers could be trained for the task.

"Putting those capacities in place," Fineberg continues, "along with adequate personal protective equipment, intensive care, and ventilators for treatment, is the second critical condition. The third condition to satisfy before a specific region's economy can safely reopen is decreasing cases to a low enough number so that if infections start to escalate, they can still be controlled. If, for example, it's down to a hundred cases in a given area, and you could contain, say 300, if you multiply 100 by three, three again, and three once more over the succeeding two weeks, all of a sudden you have 2700 cases. That's very different than if you started with 10 and had 270, a number that's still containable."

Fineberg further explains what needs to be done in an editorial published today in the *New England Journal of Medicine.* "The President says we are at war with the coronavirus," he writes. "It's a war we should fight to win. The economy is in the tank, and anywhere from thousands to more than a million American lives are in jeopardy. Most analyses of options and trade-offs assume that both the pandemic and the economic setback must play out over a period of many months for the pandemic and even longer for economic recovery. However, as the economists would say, there is a dominant option, one that simultaneously limits fatalities and gets the economy cranking again in a sustainable way."

The goal, Fineberg says, shouldn't be to flatten the curve. The goal ought to be to crush it. "China did this in Wuhan," he says. "We can do it across this country in ten weeks."

Fineberg thinks POTUS should "surprise his critics and appoint a commander who reports directly to the President." He'd carry the full power and authority of POTUS to "mobilize every civilian and military asset needed to win the war." Each governor would appoint a state commander with similar statewide authority. Fineberg outlines further steps. Make millions of diagnostic tests available. Get PPE to health care workers. Trace contacts of cases and quarantine them in now empty hotels for two weeks. Inspire and mobilize the public. After health care providers have enough, direct the USPS to deliver masks to each American family. Encourage people to wear them in public, to protect friends, neighbors, and everyone else.

To POTUS, COVID should have been a political gift. What American president has been turned out of office in a crisis? Lincoln during the Civil War? (I know, the South wanted to.) FDR during the depression, or WWII? But these men were *leaders*. They had *character*—FDR's forged by post-polio paralysis, Lincoln's by depression, perhaps brought on, in part, by knowing he was, in Edmund Wilson's words, America's "most prolific executioner."

Not to derogate the challenges of POTUS's prolonged adolescence (has it ever stopped?) but bone spurs and trying his darndest (well, maybe not) to avoid STDs during the Vietnam War while avoiding service in Southeast Asia pale by comparison.

Regarding leadership, it ain't rocket science! Give the job to any governor! On second thought, maybe not "don't-close-the-beaches" DeSantis. Or Oklahoma's Stitt—if he was a Democrat, POTUS would confer on him a nifty nickname—who tweeted a pic of his smiling and unmasked mug at a crowded restaurant. Or Kemp of Georgia, who until recently didn't know that asymptomatic patients could transmit COVID, and whose "plan" for reopening the Peach State's economy even POTUS considers daft.

It's so easy! Really! We'll give the president a little list:

1. Inspire the nation. Remind people of what we've accomplished before. Defeating fascism. Winning the Cold War. Building the most vibrant economy in world history, house of cards though it may turn out to be. Prepare us for suffering and sacrifice, cast aside divisiveness. Unify us in this patriotic cause! Read Churchill's speeches.

2. Use the Defense Production Act to its full capacity. Make gazillions of masks, testing reagents, and nasal swabs. Turbocharge testing capacity. Set a goal of increasing it across the country by two orders of magnitude.

3. Hire and train 300,000 workers from the ranks of the 26.5 million newly unemployed to trace contacts of patients with COVID. Quarantine them apart from their families in unused hotels.

4. In public, insist that everyone wears a mask. No "you can do it, you cannot do it. I don't think I'm gonna." Not anymore. Set an example! Wear one yourself!

5. Empower state and local officials to make science-based decisions on how and when to reopen the economy, guided by principles spelled out by Dr. Fineberg and other experts. Tell Americans we can't have a healthy economy without ensuring the health of the workers who are the engines of its growth. Like a just-married couple, remind us the two must go hand in hand.

I become hopeful—it would be so easy to lead, perhaps POTUS can rise to the occasion and pull it off—and then the optimism ebbs, my emotions changing like weather in the Wisconsin spring: sunny and warm one moment and cold and dreary the next.

Can I sign off without recognizing the bard's birthday? All the world's a stage, and all the men and women merely players. They have their exits and their entrances, and one man in his time plays many parts.

Oh, Lawrence Olivier, oh, Mr. President, wherefore art thou?

RAISE A GLASS WITH ME

April 24

On April 19, Steve, from Watertown, Wis., joined 80 protestors taking a Sunday constitutional around the state capitol in Madison. He wore an American flag bandanna on his head and carried a Gadsden flag inscribed with "Don't Tread on Me." Steve, who didn't want his last name known, said the extension of Governor Evers safer-at-home order had "nothing to do" with stopping the spread of COVID.

"There is an agenda throughout the world," he said, "to have a one-world government to do away with borders. To do away with nationalism and sovereign countries. And that is a huge mistake. This plays right into their playbook. Their agenda is misinformation."

Steve believes Anthony Fauci is in Bill Gates' back pocket.

Another man echoed Steve, claiming Gates owns the WHO.

"Sure seems coincidental," he said. "This is a power grab and a money grab. We got these central bankers and powerful people. People like Bill Gates. He's not satisfied with being rich. He wants control. This is all about hype and fear. People need to be able to see through the smoke of lies that they are being fed."

Signs re-enforced talking points. "No tests, no vaccine, no masks." "Mainstream media lies to you." "The government that governs least is best."

Two women carried a banner between them that read, "Bill Gates + Epstein + Fauci = vaccines."

Dimitra Anderson lives in Milwaukee. She's a professional belly dancer, Greek immigrant, and best friend of another Greek émigré I dated a few months before meeting my wife. Dimitra was clad in American flag garb from head to toe—regalia I'd never seen and hadn't known she possessed, together with her politics, which were starkly different from my former girl-friend's—and held aloft a "rebel with a cause" sign.

"I didn't choose to live in this country with no logic and to sit idle," she said. "I'm exercising my freedom. Don't tell me what to do. I turned 60 last week and my party was at Pic 'n Save with the dairyman and the meat man I've known for years," she added as her eyes grew moist. "I've lost my liberty and they can't take that away from me."

Perhaps I should have anticipated this sort of passion from a Greek, and a belly dancer to boot—though I never saw her perform—but Dimitra never hinted at it in my company.

Today, coincident with the end of the first safer-at-home decree recently extended by Gov. Evers through May 26, protestors again are amassing in Madison. Who's right? Evers or the protestors? Do both have valid points?

In Wisconsin, bars and restaurants were ordered closed on March 17 (in Eau Claire, most had shut their doors a day earlier) and the first safer-at-home directive came March 25. We've been social distancing in the Badger State for five and half weeks.

It's worked. A month ago, Wisconsin had the nation's 15th highest number of COVID cases. Now, we're 26th. In west-central Wisconsin, we're better off yet. Eau Claire County, population 104,000, has had only two new cases in the last two and half weeks. From the start of the pandemic, the tri-county area, which includes Dunn and Chippewa Counties, with a combined population of 215,000, has had only 52. Fully 70 percent of Wisconsin's cases are in four of its 72 counties—Milwaukee, Brown, Dane, and Waukesha—with the city of Milwaukee hardest hit.

In testing, Wisconsin is average: 9,779 tests per million residents, comparable to Ohio, Georgia, Nebraska, or Kentucky. As expected, harder hit states, which have bigger cities, have higher testing rates, led by New York at more than 35,000; tragically, the Empire State has had 268,000 COVID cases causing 21,000 deaths. Among the states, there's a correlation, albeit imperfect, between cases and tests. (The leader, Rhode Island, has tested 42k of its one million residents, though their COVID caseload comes in at 22nd. CVS, headquartered in a Providence suburb, has juiced the state's testing program.)

In the tri-county area of west-central Wisconsin, though we have a low COVID disease burden of 53 cases and zero deaths, we've done 3,200 tests (thanks to Mayo!) for a rate of 14,884 per million residents, slightly above the national average and half again higher than the mean of our state.

CNN ran a piece yesterday entitled, "The naïve—and reckless—rule breakers of COVID-19," which portrayed several perceived scalawags. A Washington, D.C., media consultant who attends 200 cocktail parties a year snuck in through a host's back door to a movie producer's dinner party. Food was prepared by a live-in chef and served to a group of four who sat in a garden six feet apart. A trio of real estate executives rotates houses and gets drunk together every night. Classist critique, do you think?

"I even know elderly people in the United Kingdom," the correspondent intoned, referring to her native country, "who've gone over to each other's gardens to sit six feet apart for a glass of wine."

Well!

Shouldn't we focus on what's truly irresponsible? "So supposing we hit the body with a tremendous—whether it's ultraviolet or just a very powerful light," said POTUS yesterday. "And then I said supposing you brought the light inside the body, which you can do either through the skin or some other way…"

Referring to bleach, POTUS added, "I see the disinfectant that knocks it out in a minute, one minute. And is there a way we can do something like that by injection inside, or almost a cleaning? Because you see it gets inside the lungs and it does a tremendous number on the lungs, so it would be interesting to check that."

His father died of Alzheimer's disease, which can run in families—POTUS can't read from a teleprompter; he can't pronounce hydroxychloroquine despite countless attempts; Alzheimer's patients typically are unaware of their deficits.

POTUS, please! Get thee to a neurologist!

The economic pain from the virus is all too real. People need to get back to work! Is there a middle ground between Governor Evers and the people who, as I write, are protesting his policies? (They'd expected thousands in Madison but only hundreds showed up; perhaps scores had injected disinfectant on POTUS's advice and knocked themselves out of commission.) When can Wisconsin safely reopen for business?

My father, who decades ago dabbled in oil landscapes, sometimes warns me against painting people with broad strokes of a brush. Lest I leave you thinking that all lockdown protestors need their Q'Anon fix each night before hitting the hay, let me quote Russ Lachman, 69, of La Crosse, interviewed at today's rally.

"You've got two major areas in Wisconsin that are bad: Milwaukee, probably Madison, but the rest, especially the western part of the state, there's nothing."

When can Wisconsin safely reopen for business? I agree with Mr. Lachman that it depends on the part of the state. In the southeast, it's too soon. But not only is west-central Wisconsin now a fairly safe place, it's hard to conceive of it becoming safer anytime in the upcoming year—unless we perform more tests, and masks are mandated in every indoor public space.

Any plans for the weekend? We're not islands, you know, we humans, and it's supposed to be nice. Want to have friends or family over for some wine? If you sip it outside and sit six feet apart, lift a glass for me.

COVID CAN KILL
YOU IN MANY WAYS

April 25

Nick Cordero grew up in Hamilton, Ontario. After attending Ryerson University for two years, he left to perform in the rock band Lovemethod, which released a 2003 album entitled *If You Will.*

The band broke up, and Cordero, now 41, made his way to New York. In 2009, he originated the title role in the off-Broadway musical *The Toxic Avenger.* On Broadway in 2012, he played Dennis in *Rock of Ages.* Two years later, he received a Tony nomination for Best Featured Actor in a Musical for his role in *Bullets Over Broadway.* Starring roles in *Waitress* and *A Bronx Story* followed. He and his wife have a 10-month-old son.

One week ago, his right leg was amputated, a complication of COVID, for treatment of which Cordero's been in an Los Angeles ICU since April 1, when he was sedated and put on a ventilator. When that failed to deliver enough oxygen, his doctors turned to ECMO (extracorporeal membrane oxygenation), a heart-lung machine similar to those used in cardiac surgery. Kidney failure led to dialysis. Complications from an ECMO catheter contributed to clots in his leg, blood thinners to treat the clots caused internal bleeding, and the leg had to be amputated. Now off sedation, Cordero hasn't woken up. Whether his presumed brain damage was caused by ECMO or COVID isn't clear. How did the virus wreak all of this multi-organ havoc?

"COVID can attack almost anything in the body with devastating consequences," says Yale cardiologist Harlan Krumholz. "Its ferocity is humbling and breath-taking."

When an infected person breathes or coughs, COVID can lodge in the throat or nose of someone nearby. In the mucous membranes of that nose, rich with receptors for angiotensin-converting enzyme 2 (ACE2) (COVID needs these receptors, which mark other organs for subsequent damage, to enter a cell) the virus finds a welcome home.

For up to a week, a newly infected and asymptomatic person may shed copious amounts of virus. If the immune system doesn't defeat it, COVID marches down the trachea and into the lungs, where it finds another receptive environment in microscopic air sacs called alveoli—also rich with ACE2 receptors—which exchange carbon dioxide for oxygen. As COVID replicates in the alveoli, sometimes coupled with a too-robust immune response that damages alveolar capillaries, coughing and breathlessness ensue.

Elevated levels of cytokines, molecules that stimulate inflammation, have been found in patients' blood. Some doctors believe a "cytokine storm" causes blood vessels to leak, blood pressures to plummet, clots to form, and organs to fail, until the patient dies.

"The real morbidity and mortality of this disease is probably driven by this out-of-proportion inflammatory response to the virus," says James Garfield, a pulmonologist at Temple University.

Others disagree. "There seems to have been a quick move to associate COVID with these hyperinflammatory states," says Joseph Leavitt, a Stanford ICU specialist. "I haven't really seen convincing data that that is the case." Leavitt worries that anti-cytokine drugs currently in clinical studies may blunt the immune response needed to get rid of the bug.

If not through a cytokine storm, how else does COVID injure and kill?

In Brescia, Italy, a 53-year-old woman walked into an ER with classic heart attack symptoms, a diagnosis also suggested by an EKG and elevated blood troponin, a cardiac muscle protein that leaches into the blood during such an attack. An echocardiogram showed a weak and enlarged heart. But when doctors did a coronary angiogram, her arteries were clean. COVID had invaded her heart muscle.

The cardiovascular system, replete with ACE2 receptors, offers COVID multiple targets. In a Chinese study of 416 patients, 20% had heart damage. Blood vessels are prone to clot excessively. Clots in veins can lead to pulmonary embolism, and arterial clots can precipitate a stroke or heart attack.

Last night on CNN, an emotional Anderson Cooper interviewed a young woman whose husband had recently succumbed to the virus. The couple has two young children. The man had been improving in the ICU until he suddenly coded and died. Likely, a pulmonary embolism or a clot in a coronary caused his death.

Thomas Oxley is an interventional neurologist in Manhattan. Recently, he was called to the OR to remove a clot from a 44-year-old's brain, a man who was COVID positive. As Oxley used a needle-like device to extract the clot, he saw something he'd never seen before—new clots forming around it in real time.

"We are used to thinking of 60 as a young patient when it comes to large vessel occlusions," says Eytan Raz, an assistant professor of neuroradiology at NYU Langone Medical Center. "We have never seen so many (stroke patients) in their 50s, 40s, and late 30s."

Not only do arteries have a tendency to clot, they can constrict abnormally, depriving tissues of needed blood. In the lung, they may *fail* to constrict *normally*, which may explain why some patients, despite having oxygen levels as low as Sherpas on Mt. Everest, aren't gasping for breath.

Usually, as my physiology professor taught in med school, when facing a challenge, the body is smart. In a typical pneumonia, pus-filled alveoli in part of a lung, the pulmonary arteries constrict there and shunt blood from the site. Why stop at a gas station if there's no fuel in its tanks? At this point it's hypothetical, but perhaps with COVID, in response to oxygen-starved alveoli, blood flows to them as if the air sacs are functioning normally, though there's no O2 on which to fill up. Oxygen levels become perilously low, but patients aren't aware of it.

In up to 50 percent of cases, COVID affects the kidneys, which have one of the body's highest concentrations of ACE2 receptors.

About 20 percent of COVID patients have diarrhea—sometimes it's the predominant symptom—on account of an abundance of colonic ACE2.

A "sympathetic storm" associated with severely elevated blood pressure can precipitate seizures, which may also be triggered by direct brain infection, the virus perhaps gaining entrée through the brainstem's olfactory bulb, infection of which causes the often-observed loss of smell and taste.

The pathophysiology at once fascinates and horrifies. I'm reminded of a virus from the 1980s and early 90s, until combination anti-retroviral therapy changed it from a death sentence into a chronic disease.

The last textbook I purchased, in 1994, was the *Textbook of AIDS Medicine*. Since then, for the most part, online resources have replaced books. But I can imagine, within a year, a similar 1,000-page COVID tome.

We'll be fortunate to see Nick Cordero on a Broadway stage, ever again.

Addendum: On July 5, Cordero died.

ARE RULES MADE TO BE BROKEN?

April 26

Today I had a different topic in mind, but fate had other plans. Yesterday my wife and I took a hike at Hoffman Hills, a state park half an hour west of Eau Claire. I loaded my pack with a bottle of pinot noir and two plastic cups. The night before I'd reached out to good friends, who we hadn't seen since the virus upended everyone's lives, to see if they wanted to join us.

They were keeping a low profile, my friend said. They'd love to see us, but they were concerned about seeing even their kids. He suggested a virtual happy hour. Love, he signed off. Even pre-COVID, we've been doing that—texting Love, and then our names—because we're in our 60s now, and you never know.

I'm fortunate to have wonderful friends, many of whom I've known since childhood, and this man is at the top of the list. He's the father, friend, and husband I aspire to be. We met in sixth grade, playing on a YMCA football team coached by my dad, who called my friend one of the best football players he'd coached in his 12-year career. "When I told him to do something," my dad said, "he *did* it."

Our friendship was cemented in junior high. One hot day in late May (the school lacked air conditioning) I had a bad case of poison ivy—one eye swollen shut, blisters seeping, fluid trickling down my face. In the cafeteria over lunch, I leaned back, eyes shut and head against the table. My friend went to the bathroom and soaked paper towels in cold water to lay on my face. Several times, he replaced the towels. The relief was temporary, but the gratitude has never stopped.

We sang in the choir, which was entertaining. 14-year-old boys don't stand on risers for 50 minutes without cutting up. Looking back, I feel bad for the choir teacher, but I didn't back then. When Mr. Russell got mad, his ears turned red, which made us smile.

There was a bully in choir, and he stood on the riser behind my friend. Bullies pick on people they perceive as weak. Regarding my friend, he made a mistake. Day after day, the bully provoked him. Called him sissy, and worse. "Knobbed" him on the back of the head, knuckles to the noggin', again and again.

My friend turned to him and said, "You should stop that."

When he didn't, I came up with a plan. After school, the two would fight. A would-be Don King, I promoted the bout.

The bully had a reputation as a dirty street fighter. My friend, always and ever a nice guy, had wrestled but never fought. As a 6'1", 160-pound senior lineman, he started both ways in football. Wrestling at 155 pounds, he lost just one match as a senior before dislocating his shoulder in the state sectionals. He set the all-time Eau Claire Memorial High School record for overhand pull-ups at 46, a record that stands to this day.

But that was all to come. Back then, I simply had faith in my friend. I knew he'd win.

A week later, on the banks of the Chippewa River behind the Young Men's Christian Association and egged on by a score or more junior high fight fans, few of whom thought my friend had a chance (the bully was bigger), they duked it out. The bully lunged at my friend, who parried the attack, threw him to the ground, and proceeded to pummel him. It wasn't long before the bully said, "I give." My friend got off him and walked away. The bully dragged himself and his bloody nose off the ground. He ran over and kicked my friend, who kept walking. The bully never bothered him again.

Before our hike, my wife and I were writing—she's working on a memoir about life with her son, who died six years ago, at age 19, from complications of spinal muscle atrophy—sitting at opposite ends of the kitchen table, pounding on our laptops. I was struggling to find the right words, she wanted to finish a chapter, and we didn't pull into the trailhead until close to five.

People were leaving, a previously full parking lot emptying out—vehicles remained in the overflow area—and the sun, in its glory all day, had slipped beneath the clouds. The grass was beginning to green, you had to look closely to see buds on the trees, a woodpecker rat-tat-tatted off the trail up ahead. Dressed in shorts and a t-shirt for the first time this year, I was chilled as we started out, but warmed up on the uphill trek to the observation tower on top of the ridge.

When it loomed in sight, my heart sank. A cluster of people were already there. Young men, it appeared. No surprise on such a nice day. But so much for romantic time for my wife and me.

They were older teenagers, shaggy hair, scruffy beards, but who was I to criticize? There's not much room at the top, perhaps 12-foot square. I led Monica upwind from the lads, so any COVID they might exhale would be borne away from us and over the farms patching the hardwood forest that stretched out in back of them dozens of miles.

What would happen if one of them jumped, they wondered? Sixty feet to the ground, one outcome quite certain, a conclusion on which minutes later the group agreed. I uncorked the wine, poured two glasses.

One man commanded the conversation, gesturing as he did. Nervous-like, jittery. His blond hair was disheveled, a few adolescent whiskers sprouted from his chin like blades of grass on a dune, and his dirty jeans were in danger of slipping over his scrawny hips. He turned to us, lit a cigarette, and asked, "Nice day, huh?"

"It really is," I said. "We couldn't get anyone to join us. You millennials, compared to us boomers, look at this virus a little differently."

"I guess," he said, turning back to his friends.

There were titters of laughter as they looked away, over the railing, surveying the countryside. Monica and I sipped our wine and did the same. The scenery was bland, compared to autumn, when the maples would be ablaze in red and orange and yellow. Now, from a distance, the branches were bare. The man caught our eyes again.

"Hey," he said. "I just want to give you a heads-up. I'm on the run."

I cocked my head. "On the lam from the law, you mean?"

He nodded.

"You have our full attention," said Monica, taking a step in his direction.

He cracked a grin, like a rock does to a windshield, kicked up by a semi truck. "I was drivin' the back roads," he said. "Goin' about a hundred, and I passed a sheriff and kept goin'."

"I see," I said.

"So he comes after me. I mean he's gainin', I'm goin' a hundred, but I know all of them roads, and I lost him." He took a breath. "But I'm thinking about turning myself in."

I should have said, "Good idea." Instead, I asked, "Did he get your license plate?"

The man shook his head. "He never got closer than a block. He didn't have to. My truck is well-known to them. It sorta stands out."

"Hmm," I said. "Are you well-known to them, too?" My youngest son had been a cop in Menomonie, the closest town, and I wondered if he'd made his acquaintance.

"Kinda. But I've never spent more than two nights in jail," he said, adding, "In a row."

"For fleeing, you might be looking at a month in prison," I said.

"The county jail," he corrected.

"Right," I said. He reminded me of inmates I'd seen from the Eau Claire County jail when they were taken to the free clinic for medical care. They'd had bad breaks, made dumb choices, and had untreated addiction and mental health problems. Not a true bad apple in the bunch.

"I've got relatives in California," he said. "I'm thinking of heading there."

Another idea I should have discouraged. But running from the law, in selected situations, has a certain appeal. Both times I've done it have been a blast. Apprehended by the Coast Guard for kayaking a Florida inland waterway sans lifejacket, I identified myself as David F. Wallace and made up a Madison address. And three years ago in Budapest, my wife and I were fingered for not validating our tickets when we boarded a city bus.

I know, ignorance of the law is no excuse, but the language wasn't ours and we didn't know the protocol. A local lady pled our case to the conductor, who was having none of it. "Pay the 60-euro fine," he said. "Or I'm calling the police." He followed us off the bus. We hopped back on again and he did the same. The bus moved forward before stopping at a busy intersection just before a Danube River bridge. I took my wife's hand and said, "Follow me!" We ran off the bus, through a crowd, and downstairs to the subway, emerging on a riverside walk.

The conductor, who was on the chubby side, couldn't catch us. Later, sitting outside at a bar on the banks of the Danube, the parliament illuminated across the river, the wine was especially sweet.

Perhaps in the young man, who was 18, I saw myself at that age, driving my grandpa's 1963 Plymouth Belvedere wagon, hitting a hundred on a summer day. At 18, I had a slew of tickets, though never for fleeing an officer. I take that back. A $200 ticket claimed I'd done just that. But my story was tight, and the judge let me off.

Probably good that I withheld my advice.

The man's friends bid their farewells. "Be smooth, man," said the last of the group before descending the stairs, leaving the three of us alone.

"I've decided to turn myself in," the man said. "But I'm gonna make them come up here to get me. They fucked with me, so I'm gonna fuck with them a little, too."

This time I spoke up, suggesting that this tactic wouldn't help. He shrugged his shoulders. "You're not gonna jump, are you?" I asked, adding, "I'm a doc." Too many of my patients have committed suicide—one is too many—and nothing's worse.

"No, no, of course not," he said. "Why would I do that?"

I repacked the wine and cups and shouldered the pack. "Take care," I said, extending my hand. His was the first I'd shaken in weeks—even amongst family and friends, handshakes are out and elbow bumps de rigueur—but he needed it.

Rule breaker, or rule follower? In the time of COVID, one's choices can have existential consequences. Make up our own minds or do what we're told? Does it depend on the situation? How do, how will, you decide?

LEADERS AND ABUSERS

April 27

"Mask 19," says the woman in Paris, France, to the pharmacist behind the counter. The words are a code informing the pharmacist she's being physically abused. France followed Spain's lead, to give women a lifeline out of abusive relationships.

Sad that this is necessary. But around our locked-down world, police and domestic violence hotlines are reporting a surge in victims' calls. Sheltering at home, for too many women, is anything but.

If you're not living in an abusive situation, it's hard to appreciate the dynamic. Someone is beating you up? Why don't you leave? For nine years, I had the privilege of being a director for the Bolton Refuge House, Eau Claire's domestic violence shelter, which helped me understand.

Abusers control their victims. They isolate them from friends and family, so a victim hears only the criminal. They destroy self-esteem by repeating, "No one else would want you." Beatings are followed by "honeymoon" periods where the abuser apologizes and promises it won't happen again. But the cycle continues, until the woman is either killed or manages to escape.

Determining if you're being controlled by an abuser can be harder to sort out than you might think. Abusers are bullies, but they can be charming, making their hold on you hard to dislodge. Friends who share a different perspective can be invaluable.

In *The Irish Times*, Fintan O'Toole writes that POTUS "has destroyed the country he promised to make great again. The world has loved, hated, and envied the U.S. Now, for the first time, we pity it."

The Japan Times, referring to POTUS's now-canceled daily COVID briefings ("a waste of my time," he declared) says the briefings "were bound to become all about this most limelight-loving of presidents." POTUS "made himself lead actor, director, and producer in the latest version of a reality TV show he has been playing much of his life—the omnipotent, irascible chief executive."

According to *Der Spiegel*, "nowhere in the Western world has (the pandemic) brought to light shortcomings as relentlessly as it has in the United States." The German daily says that POTUS's "disastrous crisis management has made the United States the new epicenter of the global coronavirus pandemic. The country is facing an unprecedented economic crash."

The Australian writes that POTUS "shocks with disinfectant injection musing."

Foreign leaders such as Angela Merkel, whom POTUS often maligns, usually listen politely to his inchoate ramblings in the interest of preserving the broader relationship, according to *The Guardian*. But his "ineptitude and dishonesty in handling the pandemic, which has left foreign observers as well as Americans gasping in disbelief, has proved a bridge too far. Erratic behavior, tolerated in the past, is now seen as downright dangerous. It's not just about failed leadership," says the British daily. "It's about openly hostile, reckless actions."

Beppe Severgnini is a veteran Italian author and journalist. He's traveled extensively in America, where he lived as a correspondent for *Correrre della Sera*, an Italian daily. From his home in hard-hit northern Italy, looking across the Atlantic at the U.S., Severgnini says, "When something like this happens it becomes obvious and clear to everyone that you need a wise and calm and steady hand when the sea is stormy. The sea is stormy and the captain is dancing on the deck, shouting at the wind."

If there's something god-awful with either the man you're living with or the one elected President, it may be hard to see the forest through the trees in which you're enmeshed. What would a good boyfriend look like? How should a leader act? What should he or she do?

Today New Zealand Prime Minister Jacinda Ardern said her country has defeated COVID—for now. The island nation announced the lifting of most restrictions imposed to halt the virus's spread. Schools will resume, and most businesses may open their doors.

"There is no widespread undetected community transmission in New Zealand," Ardern said. "We have won that battle. But we must remain vigilant if we are to keep it that way."

In New Zealand, population 5 million, only 19 people have perished from COVID, and the country reported just five new cases today. Ardern emphasized that new cases will continue to be found, but the number will be manageable because of scaled up contact tracing capable of making 10,000 calls a day.

The 39-year-old Ardern is the second world leader, after Benazir Bhutto, to have given birth while at her nation's helm. She's used her communications degree effectively to urge Kiwis to "be strong and be kind." (I've visited the country twice, and both seem national traits.)

Helen Clark, herself a former prime minister, says people feel that Ardern "doesn't preach at them; she's standing with them. They may even think, well, I don't quite understand why the government did that, but I know she's got our back. There's a high level of trust in her because of that empathy."

Ardern's empathy has been on frequent display during Facebook live chats that are both informal and informative. During one evening session, she appeared in an old sweatshirt after she'd just put her toddler to bed and sympathized with how alarming it must have been to hear the "loud honk" that preceded the emergency alert message informing New Zealanders that life as they knew it was temporarily over. She encourages people to consider the group with whom they're "hunkering down" as their "bubble," and to act "as though you already have COVID" toward anyone outside of it. She justifies severe policies with practical examples. People need to stay local, she says, because what if you're driving cross country and your car suddenly breaks down? According to *The Atlantic*, Ardern "may be the most effective leader on the planet."

Angela Merkel was born in 1954 in a small town in East Germany just north of Berlin. Her father, a Lutheran minister, was surveilled by the Stasi. Though a brilliant student, Merkel learned early "not to put herself in the center of things." In 1989, when the Berlin Wall fell, Merkel, who earned a Ph.D. in quantum chemistry, was working as a research scientist. (I'm impressed. In college, I, too, majored in chemistry, and I took exactly one course in quantum chemistry, where I barely eked out 20 percent—a middle C—on the final exam. I stopped reading the textbook at page seven, figuring that if those initial pages didn't register, the rest wouldn't either.)

Soon after the wall fell, Merkel left her job to join a political group. She's never publicly disclosed her reason for leaving a promising scientific career for politics, but it's postulated that, hailing from under-resourced East Germany, Merkel thought she couldn't compete with her western peers. By 2005, she was chancellor.

Her measured approach to governance succeeds in a country that reveres scientific progress—Einstein, Koch, Planck, etc—but fears charismatic leaders like the bully who took the reins of Deutschland in 1933.

Since she's from East Germany, Merkel puts a premium on freedom. On March 18, flanked by German and EU flags, she gave a televised speech that solidified her leadership, conceding that "our idea of normality, of public life, social togetherness—all of this is being put to the test as never before. Since the Second World War," she continued, "there has not been a challenge for our country in which action in a spirit of solidarity on our part was so important. I firmly believe that we will pass this test if all citizens genuinely see this as their task."

Eloquent, inspiring, and commonsense words.

If you're being abused, you deserve better—as does every American.

A FAILURE
OF IMAGINATION

April 28

"Capitalism is the worst economic system, except for all others." Churchill didn't actually speak those words, but you can imagine him doing so.

Capitalism is great at wealth generation, and with adequate adjustments and controls—progressive income tax, earned income tax credit, protections for workers, consumers, and the environment—it works quite well. Even Elizabeth Warren—my choice for president—is a capitalist.

Health care in America is a capitalist industry. I say "industry" instead of "system," because to describe American health care as the latter isn't true. In the U.S., health care players respond to economic incentives.

It's often said that America has the best health care "system" in the world. Is that accurate? True, our research and innovation are second to none.

But in 2018, 27 million Americans didn't have health insurance, up two million from the previous year. (In 2009, before Obamacare, 46 million Americans were uninsured at a given time, and 58.5 million lacked insurance at least part of that year; studies from the 2000s found that, in the richest country on earth, between 18,000 and 50,000 Americans died each year—reasons include lack of preventive care or waiting too long to treat conditions that could have been cured if evaluated earlier—because of not having insurance.)

Liberté, égalité, fraternité, say the French. In the United States—a misnomer in the POTUS era—only the first is true.

The Organization for Economic Cooperation and Development (OECD) is comprised of 36 countries, all in Europe or North America, except Mexico, Chile, and Japan. In infant mortality, the U.S. ranks 33 of 36 with 5.9 deaths per 1,000 live births. Only Vermont and New Hampshire, the top two states in this stat, match the OECD's 3.9 average. Iceland ranks first with 0.7 deaths per 1,000 births.

In life expectancy at birth, the U.S. ranks 28th at 78.6 years, just below the Czech Republic (79.1) and seven months ahead of Poland and Turkey (tied at 78.) It's worth noting that if you live to 80 in America, your life expectancy is the best in the world.

Credit Medicare!

We achieve these mediocre results despite spending 50 percent more per capita on health care than anyone else, a whopping $3.6 trillion a year, $11,000 for every man, woman, and child.

But if you want a knee replacement, or need a heart valve replacement, or an MRI, you can get it fastest in America. You'll just pay through the nose. Rather, the government or your insurance will, because these procedures, compared to talking with your family doc, are reimbursed at exorbitant rates.

Again, health care providers respond to economic incentives. Wouldn't you? If that's the "system" in which you live and work?

In northwest Wisconsin, my employer has been very profitable. The only time we ran in the red was the summer of 2017, when we adopted an awful electronic health record (EHR). (More on this Epic failure to come.)

The profitability owes a lot to our inverted pyramid. Most clinics have a large base of primary care providers and a smaller set of specialists at the top. But in Eau Claire, we have more cardiologists, orthopedists, and radiologists—more of each group—than we have internists, and the proceduralists and x-ray readers, because they rake in a ton of dough, are paid multiples of my salary.

I'm not complaining. My compensation is more than enough. And I'm a simple person, as my friends and colleagues will attest. There are only three things you can do with money—have things, do things, or give it away. Of course you can save money, too, letting you have things, do things, or give it away at a later date. You can guess my priorities; I've had a blessed life.

In 2009, as part of the Health Information Technology for Economic and Clinical Health (HITECH) Act, the federal government allocated $27 billion to encourage hospitals and providers to adopt electronic health records (EHRs). Vendors of EHRs rushed to gobble up money like pigs at a trough, developing and disseminating woefully inadequate software. Wisconsin-based Epic, if success is defined as sales, came out on top.

At a cost of $2 billion, my employer contracted with Epic for an enterprise-wide EHR. The result has been a "system" in which providers average an hour of clerical time for every hour they spend with patients. Schedulers no longer can enter orders for labs or x-rays; providers must search for and click on each one. In the past, if I wanted an EKG on a patient I was examining, I simply asked my nurse to order it. Now not only must the order be entered, if it's not entered correctly, the technician can't do the cardiogram. A recent survey of Mayo and Stanford physicians, published last month in the *Mayo Clinic Proceedings*, gave EHRs an average grade of "F."

Why is this tolerated? Because administrators love them. The "successful" EHRs were designed as billing platforms, and Epic is a billing platform par excellence. Of course this, too, adversely affects clinical care, but no matter, because the institution is awash in cash. (Pre-COVID, that is.)

Rather than a dictated note detailing a patient's narrative (the story they want told and the account doctors should want to hear), notes are cut and pasted. They go on and on ad infinitum, the documented details contributing less and less to patient care; the echo of an echocardiogram done in 2015 continues to reverberate.

The more info on the chart, the higher the allowable charge. It's not a coincidence that my personal physician, Dr. Stephen Rogers, who consistently has the highest patient satisfaction ratings in our department, dictates his charts, one of few docs here who still do.

Not only do we risk devaluing patients' histories, together with the personal traits that may forge bonds with them (there's no place in a cut-and-paste note for how the founder of a local travel agency reminds me of my beloved grandfather) the push for excessive documentation may make us worse diagnosticians.

As medical students, we're taught to chart in a SOAP format: subjective, objective, assessment, and plan. The assessment is the differential diagnosis, the various diseases the patient may have. Now, beneath mountains of data, the assessment of patients in the ER might be "chest pain." Chest pain ain't an assessment! Chest pain is the *chief complaint*, the beginning of the patient's history. Myocardial infarction, pulmonary embolism, a rupturing aortic aneurysm, pleural inflammation, bruised ribs, and much else, are among its causes.

COVID has laid bare the inadequacies of a health care "system" organized around the profit motive. Only one in 40 health care dollars is spent on public health, because where's the money to be made in *that*? When 2020 began, the national strategic stockpile held 13 million N95 masks. According to Siddhartha Mukherjee's calculations, New York and California health care workers, at the height of the crisis, used that number in 11 days. But preparation doesn't turn a profit.

There's no slack in our health care delivery system. Most of our masks, both N95s and surgical, are sourced from China. So when the Chinese supply chain went down, well, why plan for such a contingency? The market, in fact, frowns on it.

When it comes to supply chains, American medicine mirrors American business. Both operate on the just-in-time principle. Keep sufficient spare parts for tomorrow only and not further ahead. Storing more is wasteful. Inefficient. Stockholders will object.

Plan for a pandemic? Have advisors in the White House keep tabs on the possibility? Embed scientists in the Chinese CDC who could warn of a coming plague?

Not a priority. Besides, after tax cuts for POTUS's pals, the money's gone.

Small wonder we've become the epicenter of the current pandemic—a role for which we set ourselves up.

Add POTUS to the mix and stir—the most divisive president in U.S. history, at a time when we most need to be unified. POTUS may fancy himself a nationalist, but a real patriot would love the country in its entirety—rich and poor, black and white—from sea to shining sea.

COVID will amplify the creative destruction ongoing in capitalist America, and health care won't be exempt. Could something new and improved rise up from the remains? Instead of health care organized around profit, imagine a system, an actual system, which attended to the fitness of the body politic and the health and well-being of each and every American.

Just imagine, if you can.

LIFE IMITATES ART

April 29

"When leaving his surgery on the morning of April 16, Dr. Bernard Rieux felt something soft under his foot. It was a dead rat lying in the middle of the landing. On the spur of the moment he kicked it to one side and, without giving it further thought, continued on his way downstairs. Only when he was stepping forth into the street did it occur to him that a dead rat had no business to be on his landing, and he turned back to ask the door-porter of the building to see to its removal."

The reaction of the door-porter surprised him. "There weren't no rats here," he said. Dr. Rieux couldn't convince him.

That evening when he came home to his apartment, a big rat approached in the hallway, spun around, and fell on its side, its mouth spurting blood. But his wife was leaving the next day for a TB sanitarium, and Rieux gave the rat no additional thought.

More dead rats followed. Everyone in the town of Oran was talking about them. When Rieux's mother came to visit, she asked, "I say, what's this story about rats going round?"

"I can't explain it," Rieux said. "It certainly is queer...but it'll pass."

Albert Camus published *The Plague* in 1947, but he started thinking about it years earlier. In August, 1942, his doctor sent him from his native Algeria to central France to recuperate from tuberculosis. Twelve weeks later, the Allies landed in North Africa, and the Germans responded by occupying the whole of southern France, ruling from the spa town of Vichy under Petain's puppet government. Camus was cut off from his wife and mother and wouldn't see them again until the end of the war. He was also separated, in author Geraldine Brooks' words (her *Year of Wonders* is set in a seventeenth century English town ravaged by the plague), from "the privilege of writing fiction." Instead, Camus served as editor-in-chief of *Combat*, a clandestine daily, and became a hero of the intellectual resistance.

The Plague, at one level, fictionalizes the exile, illness, and separation that Camus himself had experienced. "The first thing that the plague brought to our fellow citizens was exile," says his narrator. "Being separated from a loved one... (was) the greatest agony."

Who among us hasn't, even pre-COVID, felt estranged from our world? During this time of self-exile, when we're longing for connections frayed by social distancing, it may help to revisit *The Plague*. Great fiction is endowed with eternal truths.

The rats spreading contagion in Oran symbolize the Nazis that in 1940 had overrun France. In WWII, early in the occupation, many Frenchmen shared the initial reaction of *The Plague's* Father Paneloux to the epidemic: "My brethren, you deserved it."

The priest, at the surface level of the novel, meant the suffering of the afflicted was justified, or even ordained, because of their sin.

It's an all-too-common and un-Christian response. For example, AIDS, the gay plague, according to Jerry Falwell, was the punishment gay people deserved.

With COVID, this heresy against the Great Commandment has been reinvigorated. According to Pastor John Piper, "God sometimes uses disease to bring particular judgments upon those who reject him and give themselves over to sin." A prominent Texas church sponsored a billboard that reads, "Is the coronavirus a judgment from God?" Ralph Drollinger, who leads a Bible study for members of POTUS's cabinet, says COVID is "God's consequential wrath on our nation."

If the virus has been willed by God, maybe we ought to stand down. Don't fight it. Perhaps that's our president's take.

It's a sentiment with which R.R. Reno, the editor of the Christian journal *First Things*, seems to agree. "There is a demonic side to the sentimentalism of saving lives at any cost," he writes, decrying the "ill-conceived crusade against human finitude and the dolorous reality of death."

For physicians, not only does meaning inhere in such a crusade but each morning it's why we get out of bed. Fighting "the long defeat," in the words of Paul Farmer, co-founder of Partners in Health—the non-profit's work in Haiti proved that advanced HIV treatment could be successfully administered in a resource-poor country, paving the way for the 2003 President's Emergency Plan For AIDS Relief (PEPFAR) program, which has saved millions of lives—is his *raison d'être*.

POTUS toady Pastor Robert Jeffress, the minister whose recent Easter sermon the President heard, or claimed he'd listen to, says "all natural disasters can ultimately be traced back to sin."

For a time, in the Oran of *The Plague* ("in appearance, nothing had changed") life seemed to go on as before. Then as now, the enemy was invisible, whether microorganism or pernicious idea.

"Everybody knows that pestilences have a way of recurring in the world," wrote Camus, "yet somehow we find it hard to believe in ones that crash down on our heads from a blue sky."

"The city was inhabited by people asleep on their feet," he continued, too harried in their daily routines to pay an unseen microorganism any heed. "In this respect our townspeople were like everybody else, wrapped up in themselves."

Denial is widespread. When the door-porter at Rieux's building takes ill, the doctor recognizes the tell-tale signs of plague, but persuades himself that "the public mustn't be alarmed, that wouldn't do at all." The mayor "is convinced it's a false alarm." When a bureaucrat wants the spreading contagion not to be identified as such but instead as "a special type of fever," Rieux overrules him, finally accepting reality.

After a youthful flirtation, Camus abandoned communism. Religion couldn't save him—no way were epidemics and other catastrophes divinely ordained—and he'd witnessed and fought Fascism up close. Life was absurd in the sense that the circumstances in which you find yourself, often enough, simply occur.

What's not absurd is how you choose to respond. Moral persons—the commoners described by George Eliot, in the final paragraph of *Middlemarch*, as having "lived faithfully a hidden life"—look at their situations clear-eyed, decide the correct course, and follow through.

For Camus, heroism itself is suspect. One should perform the moral act, without regard for accolades either on earth or from a God in the sky. It's not by chance that he casts a mousy clerk as the embodiment of resistance to evil occupiers, be they bacilli, Nazis, or oppressive ideologies.

The author finds humankind more good than bad. Failure to act appropriately he chalks up to inertia or ignorance, something all the more important, in the run up to the November election, for people on one side of the political divide to remember about those who don't share their sensibility. Humans, Camus believed, are better than you might think. As the character Tarrou puts it, "You just need to give them the opportunity."

Rambert is a journalist separated from his wife in Paris when Oran closes its gates. He implores Rieux to write a pass for him out of the city but later puts aside his selfish desires and identifies with the "bubble" (to use Jacinda Ardern's term) of comrades within the walled city who are at war with the plague.

Like his creator, Rieux eschewed grand philosophies. "Weary of the world in which he lived," the doctor could only offer "some feeling for his fellow men," and was "determined for his part to reject any injustice or compromise."

"It may seem a ridiculous idea," he says, "but the only way to fight the plague is with decency."

TECHNOLOGY: FRIEND OR FOE?

April 30

In 1997, Arundhati Roy won the Booker Prize for her debut novel, *The God of Small Things*. Since then, she's worked mostly as a journalist and political activist. COVID, she says, "has made the mighty kneel and brought the world to a halt like nothing else could. Our minds are still racing back and forth, longing for a return to 'normality,' trying to stitch our future to our past and refusing to acknowledge the rupture. But the rupture exists."

"Historically," Roy continues, "pandemics have forced humans to break with the past and imagine their world anew. This one is no different. It is a portal, a gateway between one world and the next. We can choose to walk through it, dragging the carcasses of our prejudice and hatred, our avarice, our data banks and dead ideas, our dead rivers and smoky skies behind us." (Roy lives in India.) "Or we can walk through lightly, with little luggage, ready to imagine another world."

So today, at her suggestion, let's walk through a portal. Neither the rabbit hole emptying into Wonderland nor the wardrobe leading to Narnia, this more humdrum portal opens onto the future practice of medicine.

On April 21, I discussed how patients weren't presenting to the hospital for even life-threatening emergencies—myocardial infarctions down by nearly 40 percent, referrals for stroke more than halved, patients with appendicitis not presenting till long after appendices burst. The hospital, many seem to think, is scarier than a heart attack, paralysis, or septic shock; dying less frightening than dialing 911.

I've also spoken of the psychological retrenchment the virus has wrought, a withdrawal into oneself. And while many are eager to break free from sheltering at home, others have become comfortable within their domiciles. The elderly have adapted best. They're at highest risk for bad COVID outcomes, a warning they heard often and took to heart. It's the same demographic that most frequently seeks medical care, particularly in my specialty, where 80 percent of my practice is 65-plus.

In my office, patients aren't showing up. In our department, fill rates for appointments are under 50 percent.

According to Kaiser Health News, "many health insurers foresee strong profits," because the falloff in claims for non-COVID care exceeds claims for patients who have COVID. The credit rating agency Moody's has looked at a range of pandemic outcomes from mild to severe and concludes that under the most likely scenarios health insurers will stay profitable.

In a paper published two weeks ago, the Radiology Society of North America anticipates a 50 to 70 percent drop in imaging volumes over at least the next three to four months.

As of next week, five nurses in our department are being furloughed without pay for four weeks. (The work has been sufficiently stressful for more than five to have volunteered.) Perhaps doctors and nurses aren't as essential as we had thought.

Decreased demand for services will lead to changes in health care delivery, to which patients will react, causing further adaptations by providers, which will further modify patients' behaviors, an action-reaction cycle eventually yielding a new status quo.

Videoconference appointments are in vogue; the website *The Medical Futurist* applauds this option to "bring health care to patients, rather than the other way around." The site further recommends digital stethoscopes and otoscopes and portable EKG monitors that would share data remotely with docs. The site says these innovations, which shift the point of care to patients, ought to become common.

Good idea? Disclaimer: As a digital immigrant rather than a digital native (I shouldn't use this as an excuse, my father would say) I'm neither a technophile nor an "early adapter" of new technologies; my son, a considerate and competent millennial, set up my blog and showed me how to upload— not download, he politely pointed out—pics to the site.

Psychologists and neuroscientists say the distortions and delays inherent in video communication can end up making people feel anxious and even more isolated and disconnected than they already do. The pixelated images, the scientists say, confound perception and scramble social cues.

Jeffrey Golde, of Columbia Business School, has been teaching his leadership class via Zoom for a month. "I've noticed, not only in my students, but also in myself, a tendency to flag," he says. "It gets hard to concentrate on the grid and it's hard to think in a robust way."

UN interpreters report similar feelings of fogginess and alienation when they interpret by video, and studies on video psychotherapy indicate that the modality causes fatigue and discomfort in both patients and therapists.

Why?

Human emotion is expressed by minute contractions of facial muscles, particularly around the mouth and eyes, which are too subtle for a screen to display. Via video, we're confused by our conversational partner's non-verbal cues, triggering anxiety, stress that may barely register, though by dialogue's end we feel drained.

When we're talking with an acquaintance, an old-fashioned face-to-face chat, our expressions, without our conscious awareness, mimic our friend's. The result is empathy, shown and received. If we don't embody empathy, or if it can't be perceived, we miss out on the kind of connection that could have occurred. Still less can true communion, which gives such pleasure, take place.

Which is worse? What's more tragic? A doctor without empathy, or a doctor whose empathy can't be discerned?

According to IT professor Sheryl Brahman, "In-person communication resembles videoconferencing about as much as a real blueberry muffin resembles a packaged blueberry muffin that contains not a single blueberry but artificial flavors, textures, and preservatives. You eat too many and you're not going to feel very good."

Four times I traveled to Haiti with Mayo medical teams. In 2015, when the program was discontinued, Mayo proposed video grand rounds to replace our physical presence in Port-au-Prince. Our Haitian colleagues declined the offer.

The organization hasn't supported doctors and nurses who want to travel to COVID hot spots, instead suggesting we make ourselves available by video to hospitalists in those regions. If there's any interest, I'll be surprised.

Mayo's 2030 strategic goal is for video appointments to comprise at least 50% of patient visits. I pray that this initiative won't succeed. If it does, I'll work elsewhere.

How will medicine look in a decade? I hope it's leaner, more focused on the necessary. Successful hospitals and clinics will offer exceptional care at a reasonable value, and patients will feel cared for.

Besides, how can a doctor examine a patient by video? As Dr. Jack Wishart told Dr. Terry Borman, who relayed the message to me, "Never underestimate the value of the laying on of hands."

DEAR POTUS:
CHINA IS WINNING

May 1

May Day, May Day! There's a cruise ship stuck off the California coast! The passengers and crew have COVID! I don't want them to dock, disembark, whatever, because if they do, my numbers will go up!

POTUS spoke those words, more or less, while visiting the CDC on March 6. How are his numbers now?

Today the U.S. surpassed 1.1 million COVID cases, one third of the known burden in the world, and U.S. deaths now exceed 65,000, 27 percent of the global toll. In large part because of POTUS's dereliction, the U.S. has become the pandemic's epicenter. Worse, we're positioned to stay there for some time.

Each day over the last six, we've averaged 28,000 new COVID infections. In the past two, we've added, on average, 2,300 daily deaths to the virus's toll. While cases and deaths in New York have diminished, other regions have picked up the proverbial slack. On a graph, if you plot cases or deaths against time, the lines go straight up. By contrast, Germany, population 83 million, reported 322 new cases and nine more deaths today.

For decades Donald McNeil has covered infectious diseases for the *New York Times*, including AIDS, Ebola, malaria, SARS, and swine and bird flu. April 29, on NPR, he described American social distancing as a "giant garden party" compared to China and Italy, which helps explain why the virus is flourishing in the United States. "China," he says, "didn't reopen until they had zero new infections a day."

The Chinese took the outbreak seriously, which meant prioritizing contact tracing. According to McNeil, the average case has 45 contacts. Twenty-eight thousand cases a day times 45 contacts per case = 1.26 million contacts a day, an impossible number for public health workers to call. But to staunch an epidemic, it's imperative, as MPH students learn in their first month of school.

China did the impossible, McNeil said. "They caught the wind," stopping a fast-moving pandemic in its tracks. "We're reluctant to follow China, but they did it. They did it brutally, but brilliantly."

The Chinese government searched for the virus relentlessly. If you tested positive, you went straight into isolation, not back with your families. "Chinese people love their families just as much as Americans love their families," McNeil said. "But when it became clear that it was saving the lives of their families, I mean, yes, some of them were forced in…chucked into the backs of ambulances by policemen. But that was not the norm. The norm was you were told, 'Please come with us to the shelter. You will have food. You will have medical care. And in three weeks, if you're good to go back home, we're going to test you, make sure you're okay, and then you can go back home.'" The vast majority complied. McNeil estimates that this "brutal" policy may have saved 10 million lives.

If CNN's Chris Cuomo had isolated himself in such a facility instead of his basement, his wife and son would be virus-free.

In the last six weeks, America has lost more than 30 million jobs, an economic calamity unprecedented in our history. Restaurants and bars have been decimated. Spending on travel and leisure has shrunk to near zilch. Retail spending has fallen off a cliff. Car sales have plummeted, housing starts have stopped, and supply chain disruptions have impaired manufacturing.

Bayard Winthrop is the CEO of American Giant, an online apparel company based in San Francisco whose Carolina factories make hoodies and flannel shirts. After the shutdown, he told his fabric suppliers he had to put purchases on hold.

"I don't think people have yet fully digested how bad this is going to be for the economy," he said. "If wallets start to really close up, it's a different scenario" (from a V-shaped economic blip.)

Today China announced 12 new cases of COVID. Their death toll is unchanged at 4,663. Chinese factories have reopened, though life, because of the psychology suggested by Winthrop, is not yet normal.

But their collective psyche is China's major concern, because government has done its job. It's safe, safe as it can reasonably be, to work in a factory, shop in a mall, or eat in a restaurant. Chinese citizens merely need to convince themselves.

Contrast this with the United States, where a dismal response to COVID has worsened economic suffering. (As a possible metaphor for our future economies, we have more than 15,000 patients with COVID in intensive care, while China has 38.) "Leadership" in Washington is stuck on square one.

Universal masking in public buildings should long since have been a national priority, but POTUS's vice won't even wear one inside the most famous clinic in the land. Doesn't he know that his mask protects others, including vulnerable patients? Aren't Christians supposed to care? Is he too macho to put one on? (His wife's assertion that he didn't know about Mayo's policy is literally incredible.) Come on, Mr. Pence! Real men wear masks!

A chance to educate, an opportunity for leadership, and perhaps prevent contagion by a lethal disease: all were squandered.

Is it possible for Pence to stand up to his boss? Put a bug in Fauci's ear, suggests Andy Borowitz. Have the good doctor tell Pence that a mask will protect him from women, so he won't be afraid of being alone with one in a room, though the women I've spoken to tell me he needn't fret.

Don't you love irony? POTUS went out of his way to wage a trade war with China. But the Chinese outsmarted him. They simply shifted the battle-ground, where they're beating our butts.

HUDDLED MASSES, YEARNING TO BREATHE FREE

May 2

On April 28, POTUS ordered meat processing plants not to close. According to the White House, "closures threaten the continued functioning of the national meat and poultry supply chain, undermining critical infrastructure during the national emergency. Given the high volume of meat and poultry processed by many facilities, any unnecessary closures can quickly have a large effect on the food supply chain."

John Tyson and his eponymous foods had the dinero for full-page ads in the Sunday *Times* and the *Washington Post*, though he couldn't come up with the cash to provide PPE for workers at his plants.

"As pork, beef and chicken plants are being forced to close, even for short periods of time, millions of pounds of meat will disappear from the supply chain," the ad said. "As a result, there will be limited supply of our products available in grocery stores until we are able to reopen our facilities that are currently closed. Millions of cattle, pigs and chickens will be euthanized because of slaughterhouse closures, limiting supplies at supermarkets."

"We're working with Tyson," said POTUS as he announced his executive order, to "solve any liability problems."

Wisconsin Senator Ron Johnson agrees. "I'm very sympathetic to (POTUS) pulling the Defense Production Act to make sure America has an adequate supply of food."

As of April 29, at least 3,300 U.S. meatpacking workers, the majority of whom are immigrants, have contracted COVID and at least 20 have died.

Recently, outbreaks at a pair of Green Bay processing plants have driven the biggest surge of COVID infections in the state. As of yesterday, cases in Brown County, home to Green Bay, stood at 1,175, doubling in a week. Green Bay Mayor Eric Genrich says POTUS is "turning his back on reality and he's turning his back on the workers who live this reality every single day." Genrich finds the President's executive order to give "meat packing conglomerates legal carte blanche in the middle of a pandemic" "reprehensible and indefensible. It's reckless and it's dangerous and it speaks to this President's complete and total inability to relate to or care about regular people here in Green Bay."

Of course POTUS's shtick is all about "relating to and caring about regular people"— unless they're undocumented, or live with someone who is: the people who process his bacon, pick grapes in his vineyard, or hang sheetrock in his hotels.

"It's not every day that the shutters of a mansion fall away and a flood of light illuminates each dark room," says essayist, actor, and Irish immigrant Maeve Higgins about COVID's consequences.

There are 4.5 million U.S. immigrants who pay taxes without official authorization, Higgins explains, using individual taxpayer identification numbers (ITINs) for the purpose. In California alone, this group pays $3 billion in state and local taxes each year. The $2 trillion CARES Act singled out people using ITINs as the only taxpayers not eligible for government aid. Moreover, if an ITIN-tax filer lives with a legal citizen, which applies to 16.7 million Americans in these "mixed-status" families, the citizens, too, are ineligible. Explains Doug Rand, a senior fellow at the Federation of American Scientists, "If a U.S. citizen, permanent resident, or anyone else with a social security number files their tax return along with anyone who doesn't have a social security number, then nobody in that household will get an emergency cash payment."

To redress this situation, some Democrats in Congress have co-sponsored a bill entitled the "Leave No Taxpayers Behind Act."

Don't hold your breath.

Lest anyone think this provision of the CARES Act was a congressional oversight, an exception was carved out for military families. Lawmakers knew what they were doing. Kentucky's Rand Paul, a physician, argued for this proviso on the Senate floor.

"If you want to apply for money from the government through the child tax credit program," Paul said, "then you should have to be a legitimate person...It has nothing to do with not liking immigrants. It has to do with saying, taxpayer money shouldn't go to non-people."

Hippocrates is rolling over in his grave, screaming "what's happened to my beloved profession? How did this doctor lose his moral compass?"

A San Diego family of five exemplifies the injustice. Miriam and her three children are citizens, but because her husband uses an ITIN, none will receive stimulus checks. "We have been filing taxes every single year for 15 years," she says. "We have paid our share and done everything we can. Our hope is that...showing we are upstanding citizens may help one day if there is a path to citizenship. And now we're in this position. It's a nationwide crisis; we feel we're being punished for doing the right thing."

In a country built upon the backs of slaves, treating some workers as at once essential and disposable is nothing new. Nor is scapegoating immigrants in times of crisis, public health or otherwise. In the 1830s, Irish immigrants were stigmatized as bearers of cholera, and TB in the late 1800s was dubbed the "Jewish disease."

Medical anthropologist Anahi Viladrich says "the systematic exclusion of immigrants is parallel with the systematic exploitation of immigrants." In

1911, the Dillingham Commission, a bipartisan investigation into immigration, concluded "the Mexican…is less desirable as a citizen than as a laborer," setting the tone for the subsequent century. After filling wartime labor shortages, Mexicans were forcibly removed from the country when they were no longer required. During the depression, more than 1 million Mexicans were deported.

1954's Operation Wetback was the biggest mass deportation of undocumented workers in U.S. history. Military-style tactics—along with portraying Latinos as dirty, disease bearing, and irresponsible—removed 1.3 million Mexicans from the United States. Each week in Chicago, three planeloads of Mexicans were flown back to their native land. In Texas, immigrants were crammed onto boats described as slave ships, while others died of sunstroke and disease while in custody.

According to migration scholar Nicholas DeGenova, "It is precisely their distinctive legal vulnerability, their putative 'illegality' and official exclusion, that inflames the irrepressible desire and demand for undocumented migrants as a highly exploitable workforce—and thus insures their enthusiastic importation and subsequent incorporation" into that force, as long as they remain "essential."

To the economy, that is.

I searched in vain for some tidbit, some measly scrap, anything to indicate that POTUS, while forcing plants to keep processing meat, might attend to the safety of the immigrants who work within—masks, social distancing mandates, something—but alas, nil. If these immigrants were allowed to vote, they wouldn't mark their ballots for him or Dr. Paul.

Cruise ships, nursing homes, aircraft carriers, prisons, and processing plants are viral incubators from which outbreaks break out into the greater society. In this pandemic, in our highly interconnected world, one man's sickness imperils everyone else. Can't POTUS see it? Can't his Vice? Will someone please lift the scales from their eyes?

BUY STUFF, PLEASE!

May 3

"The stock market is not the economy," Paul Krugman said recently. Then he tried to explain how stocks, in the wake of job losses in the last six weeks of more than 30 million, had their best month since 1987.

What else could an investor buy? Last week, 10-year Treasury yields dropped to 0.6 percent. For inflation-adjusted earnings, their yield was *minus* 0.5 percent.

Why are yields low, Krugman asked? Because interest rates are low. And why are interest rates low? Because the Fed expects the U.S. economy will stay depressed for years to come. This translates to continued easy money, a good thing for stocks.

Got it?

Me, neither.

But a disconnect between stock prices and job losses isn't unusual. How often does a corporation slash jobs and then watch its stock rise?

According to Marx, the exploitation of workers, which includes treating them as if expendable, lets capitalism thrive. In a capitalist society, power accrues to capital, but as long as workers get a fair shake, or think they do, revolutions can be kept at bay. Historically, anger feeding revolutions against capitalist countries is often calamitous for bourgeoisie and proletariat alike—something people with beaucoup capital should bear in mind.

At West Point, Al Dunlop excelled in boxing but not academics. In 1968, after completing his military service, he married Judy Stringer, of Eau Claire, Wis. He went into the paper industry and eventually became CEO of Lily-Tulip, maker of paper cups.

In 1994, Dunlop was named CEO of Scott Paper Co., where he promptly eliminated 11,000 jobs, a third of the payroll, before selling the company 15 months later for a nifty profit.

"I'm a superstar in my field, much like Michael Jordan in basketball and Bruce Springsteen in rock 'n roll," Dunlop wrote in his memoir.

"Chainsaw Al"—also dubbed "Rambo in Pinstripes" after he posed with pistols and ammunition belts—moved on to Sunbeam, where news of his hiring caused a 60 percent bump in its stock. He shuttered factories and fired half of the company's 12,000 employees. 20 months later, Sunbeam's stock had quadrupled.

Then it tanked. Less than two years after he arrived, Dunlop was canned. In 2001, Sunbeam filed for bankruptcy. For devising illegal accounting schemes to hide Sunbeam's troubles, the SEC banned him for life from serving as a public company official, and tacked on a $500,000 fine.

Five hundred grand! Talk about steep! (In 2002, Dunlop was worth $100 million.) But at Mayo-Eau Claire, perhaps we should be thankful the SEC let him off cheap, because a few years later, he and his wife gave $5 million to fund the Al and Judy Dunlop Cancer Center.

Dunlop died last year. His wife Judy survives him.

Back to stocks. At some level, they reflect earnings, and people have to spend on products or services for profits to be generated. What are the prospects?

For the most recent quarter, GDP dropped at an annualized 4.8 percent rate. But because the WHO didn't declare COVID a pandemic until March

11, and lockdown measures didn't begin until the following week, projections for GDP in the current quarter are much worse. The $64,000 question—$21 trillion, really—is the duration of the downturn.

No one knows, but according to McKinsey and Company, based on recent data, 36 percent of Americans expect an economic rebound within two to three months. Generation Z— who've reached adulthood in the last decade and are the youngest demographic able to vote—is most optimistic, perhaps because of living the least. 45 percent of Gen Z expects a quick turnaround. Compared to Americans, Europeans are pessimistic, while the Chinese express more confidence.

Few economists are as sanguine about short-term prospects for the United States. Why the dissonance?

Rather than believing we've stepped through a portal into a new era, we yearn, to paraphrase Arundhati Roy, to stitch our present to our past. A new world imagined, after all, is the stuff of science fiction. We'll get through this together—the slogan of a new Samsung commercial—suggests someday we'll leave COVID behind. Back to the future, as it were.

In general, Americans are a hopeful lot. To step on a boat, wave goodbye to the old world, and sail to an unknown land, you had to be.

The American enlightenment, which Benjamin Franklin exemplified, was an optimistic offspring of its European parent, a phenomenon discussed in my solitary peer-reviewed scientific article, "Influences of American Philosophy and History on the Practice of American Medicine," published a quarter century ago in *Mayo Clinic Proceedings*. I argued that the western frontier, coupled with this forward-looking enlightenment strain—where tomorrow would always be better than today—produced a uniquely activist medical culture in the United States. "Don't just stand there, do something!"—as American as apple pie—might not be seen that way across the pond. Instead, a French doctor might implore, "Don't just do something; please, stand still."

Unsurprisingly, the White House Council of Economic Advisors believes the glass is half full. In the recent quarter, despite "particularly sharp annualized declines on health care services (-18%), transportation (-29%), recreation (-32%), and food services and accommodations (-30%)," and "particularly steep" declines in spending on automobiles and parts (-33%), "the United States is in a strong position to recover *as the public health threat recedes.*" (Italics mine.)

Compared to China, for instance, the threat isn't receding at all. In the last twenty-four hours, China has recorded two new cases of COVID and no new deaths, while we're at 23,665 and 961.

COVID, say POTUS's economists, has "led to a whole-of-government response to bridge the current gap between a historically strong economy and the coming economic recovery." Clearly intended as a hopeful aside but sounding more like a cautionary note, they add that "when consumer confidence reached a 20-year high" (in 2019) "elevated consumer spending accounted for roughly 80 percent of real GDP growth." In the United States, compared to any other country, consumer spending will be key to our recovery, because our economy depends more on it.

But data published yesterday by the World Economic Forum don't support this rosy forecast. Over the next two weeks Americans expect to spend less than half their usual on consumer electronics, personal and pet-care services, fitness and wellness, furnishings and appliances, vehicle purchases, gasoline, hotels and resorts, foot ware, jewelry, and apparel. Spending on ambulatory health care is also projected to be down a full 50 percent.

The Chinese, in contrast, plan to spend more in nearly all categories. But they waged war on the virus, a knock-down-drag-out war, which decimated the killer's ranks, while POTUS tweets "LIBERATE MICHIGAN!"— currently number three in the U.S. in COVID deaths—a state where Dr. Birx worries aloud if protestors egged on by our president will carry the virus home to their elderly folks.

One month after the 9/11 terrorist attacks, President George W. Bush said, "The American people have got to go about their business." Go shopping, he said.

And they did. Will it be that easy, this time around?

DIVERSIONARY TACTICS

May 4

"Did you see where my ball came down?" I asked the girls in charge of refreshments, the beer and pop, as they sat in their carts. My golf ball, after slamming into a tree, had disappeared.

The three young women, two in one cart and the third in another, were parked not far from the tree that had been whacked by my ball. Erik, my son and golfing buddy, thought one girl was training a second, while I figured the third, on a warm and sunny day, simply wanted to ride around. After I'd declined a Miller Lite, Bud Light, Coors Light, Mich Light, and a Summer Shandy, like a pitcher shaking off a catcher, a girl fished deep in the cooler and came up with a Leinie's Original.

"I think it landed next to the tree," she said, correctly.

We were playing the fifth hole at Lake Hallie Golf, which runs along the Chippewa River. The wind shivered the river's surface as it gusted upstream. A woman wearing a wetsuit carved turns on water skis. The boat spun a 180, whipping her wide of the wake.

In Wisconsin, it may be mid-May before you can comfortably golf in a t-shirt and shorts, and doing so on the fishing opener felt like a gift. Erik powered his second shot on the par-4 hole onto the green, where it blazed past the pin, rocketed up an embankment, and smacked a wooden post, bouncing the ball back toward the pin. I let out a whoop.

"Better to be lucky than good," Erik said.

On the previous tee, a man with a week's growth of white whiskers tended a tripod on which was set a spotting scope.

"I'm the eagle guy," he said.

"You get an eagle on every hole?" I asked.

"Yup."

And there she was, as I gazed through the scope, perched on her nest high up in a pine.

The first hole began normally—green grass, budding trees, obese young men driving carts, my tee shot shanking into the woods—until we reached the green, where Erik informed me the pin—encircled by Styrofoam, an inch or so lower than the grass—had to stay put.

Ah, yes.

The virus.

The eighth hole follows Lake Hallie's shore. Fishing boats silently plied the water—no gas-powered motors are allowed on the lake—and canoeists and kayakers glided past, the sun glinting off paddles. Across the lake, a willow's lime-colored branches swayed in the wind. In the renaissance of spring, willow trees show the way.

"What are your three favorite outdoor memories?" Erik asked.

He's like this, posing unexpected questions, and listening to my response. I mentioned the first three that came to mind, including our second trip to Yellowstone, when Erik, now 24, was 17. We'd backpacked into a meadow and camped next to a creek. Erik was reading in the tent, I was boiling water for freeze-dried spaghetti, and when I glanced up...a bull elk. Head down, munching grass, seemingly oblivious to my presence, he moseyed toward me. I kept an eye on the elk, tiptoed to the tent, and whispered for Erik to take a peek. He poked his head out of the tent, glanced at the elk, and turned to me.

"Cool," he said.

The three of us spent an hour and a half in close company, the elk eating his supper while we enjoyed ours.

Spending time with my son and finding more balls than I lose add up to a good day of golf. In the latter category I ended up minus two, but three and a half hours with Erik was the best. Time together is precious. His fiancé is great, and he's working on an MBA; if your child is twenty-something, you know what I mean.

I played the first six holes on the back nine at 43. To card a 60, I had to play the last three holes—par 3, 4, and an over-500-yard 5—in 17 strokes.

Nearly impossible.

"You just have to play your age," he said.

"For nine holes," I said.

Erik smiled.

But then on 16, my tee-shot found its way onto the green and I two-putted for par. On the 17th, however, I dribbled my drive off the box and hit my next shot into a tree.

"Don't you love golf?" Erik asked.

"Yeah," I said.

"You've set a record for most trees hit with the ball dropping straight down."

Agreed, again. Erik hit an approach shot into an oak, banging from branch to branch before being spat out onto the green.

"Give me a break," I said.

Though sand on the course is scarce, my next shot found a trap. Sans rake to smooth over the clefts, the bunker was pocked like an acne-scarred face, as if each divot—I added two of my own—was a reminder of what COVID had taken away. I carded a snowman plus one on the par-four hole.

Fifty-five strokes, one hole to go. A par was too hopeful to even contemplate. But I'm 61. Perhaps I could shoot my age. On the back nine.

I wound up and tried to wallop my ball, which killed snakes maybe 80 yards. But then, for the first time in years, perhaps the first time in my life, I hit three decent irons in a row, putting me close enough, on my fifth shot, to chip onto the green.

Like a disapproving parent, an uphill putt stared me down. I got in position, practice putted once, and stroked the ball. The line seemed okay, but it wasn't enough. But the ball kept rolling, and rolling some more, until, perilously close to the pin, it slowed down dramatically, turned over one final time, and fell into the cup. Partway into it. Perhaps 10 feet, the putt seemed 20.

"Good way to end it," said Erik, extending his elbow, a COVID handshake.

A former high school golfer, Erik spots me a stroke and a half a hole. I shot 117, whereas Erik thought he was at ninety or less. (I'm an internist; he's working on an MBA, not studying to be a CPA; let's just say that with my handicap, the match was close.)

At the Dairy Queen, our post-golf tradition, a line of cars for takeout snaked into the street. Wait in line? Yes, we concurred. Twenty minutes later, I ordered our usual, a vanilla cone for him and chocolate for me. Next door, we commandeered an empty picnic table outside a Laundromat.

Erik licked his cone. "You know," he said, "Anissa (his fiancé) and I were talking the other day, and we both agreed that when it comes to parents, we did pretty well."

There are times when, even with COVID, all is right with the world.

WHAT ARE WE AFRAID OF?

May 5

The day after we'd golfed, I got an email from Bighorn Anglers, in Fort Smith, Mont., from whom Erik and I, seven years earlier, after eating supper with the elk, had rented a drift boat. For two days we'd floated the Bighorn River, casting flies for rainbow trout and hooking a few. I haven't been back since, and I don't remember hearing from the fly shop in the interim.

The park service opened the boat ramps on the Bighorn yesterday, the email said, but only to Montana residents. The Crow Tribe, through whose land the river flows, will grant access to non-residents, but only if they've self-quarantined 14 days in the state, a policy reinforced by Montana's governor; i.e., don't come here to fish.

The rationale is all too human: we don't have ours so don't give us yours, converse of the famous axiom. Large but sparsely populated Montana has suffered merely 457 COVID cases causing only 16 deaths.

Dillingham, Ak., population 2,400, sits on Bristol Bay's shore. Several times, my buddies and I have flown from Anchorage to the community, accessible only by boat or by plane. From Dillingham, we hop on a float plane and fly into the wilderness, where we raft, camp, and fish.

Bristol Bay is home to the world's largest spawning run of sockeye salmon, 50 million a year. The sockeye sustain a diverse ecosystem. Bears eat salmon, osprey and eagles prey on their remains, trout and grayling feed on salmon eggs and decaying flesh. One day on a Bristol Bay tributary, my friend Steve and I weaved our raft through a stream section and counted eight grizzly bears. Walking up a feeder creek, maybe a meter wide, the red salmon were stacked like a cord of wood. I reached down and grabbed two by the tail, one in each hand, held them aloft before putting them back.

Though recreational fishing aids the local economy, Dillingham depends on its commercial fishery. The sockeye are due in at the end of the month. Alaska has had 370 COVID cases and nine deaths, while the Bristol Bay region has yet to see a case. (On the Kuskokwim delta 170 miles north, Bethel reported a single case a month ago, the only evidence of contagion in southwest Alaska thus far.)

According to Andy Wink, executive director of the Bristol Bay Regional Seafood Development Association, "Thousands of fishermen travel from 48 states to work in the fishery." For their brawn and work ethic, boat captains prize men from Wisconsin and Minnesota.

Dillingham Mayor Alice Ruby doesn't want them to come. "We cannot foresee ANY plan," she wrote, "that would avoid a significant impact to our community," which has only 16 hospital beds.

But Alaska Gov. Mike Dunleavy considers commercial fishing essential. Sort of. Would-be fishermen, as in Montana, must self-quarantine 14 days after they arrive in the state.

This morning, I got an email from Hawaiian Airlines. I trained in Honolulu and retain a special affection for the islands, to which I'm fortunate to often return.

"With almost all of our fleet still grounded due to Hawaii's quarantine restrictions," wrote the CEO, "we are focusing on how we can contribute to the well-being of our communities and our guests."

Hawaii, population 1.5 million—621 cases and 17 deaths—emphasizes health and safety, sometimes to a frustrating and even exasperating degree. Omnipresent speed bumps are more than literal. Each year vehicles must pass a multi-point inspection. Over the two years my ex-wife and I lived in Honolulu, we owned five cars costing a cumulative $2,200; you can guess the quality associated with such lavish expenditures; for one of these beaters to be certified safe to drive could have been, well, problematic. The radiator of a pea-green Corona (Dear Toyota: Want to bring the model back?) required more water than the engine sucked gas, but the wagon managed to qualify, while how the Datsun passed muster (it wouldn't back up) was tougher yet to figure out.

On the northwest coast of the Big Island, I once ignored a "No trespassing" sign at the Waipio Valley trailhead in place because of a Dengue Fever outbreak in the valley below, and was escorted back uphill by a ginormous Hawaiian in a pickup truck.

Anyway.

Hawaii's two-week quarantine will last until at least the end of the month. Gov. David Ige says that while other states may have the same requirement, only Hawaii is enforcing it.

"Quarantine means you stay in your room," Ige says. "You're not allowed to leave the room. When visitors understand what that is and that we'll enforce it, we're pretty confident that they'll choose not to be here."

That tourism accounts for over a fifth of Hawaii's economy, the highest percentage in the country, doesn't seem to be part of his calculus.

Last week, New Mexico Gov. Michelle Lujan Grisham invoked the state's never-before-used Riot Control Act to lock down Gallup, a town of 22,000 in the northwest part of the state. Though Gallup doesn't fall within the boundaries of the Navajo Nation (2,373 cases, 73 deaths) it's a regional hub for Navahos and nearby pueblos of other tribes. Native Americans comprise only 11 percent of New Mexico's population but account for 53 percent of its infections with COVID.

National Guardsmen patrol the roads into Gallup, stationed on the exit ramps off the interstate, where they turn back anyone driving toward town. The Navajo worry about their citizens bringing the virus back to the reservation after shopping in Gallup, while city residents complain about Native Americans crowding into grocery stores.

Both groups are pleased with the lockdown.

In the nearby town of Grants, Mayor Martin Hicks blames the Navajo for spreading disease.

"We didn't take it to them, they brought it to us," he said. "So how are we going to spread it amongst them when they're the ones that brought it to us?"

You got it, you keep it, don't give it to us. When travel is restricted to a city or state, how much does fear, instead of concern for the locale's health, drive the decision? Fear of the other, or of COVID-19?

DRUGS FOR COVID: HYPE VS. REALITY

May 6

"Clinicians are under tremendous stress," says Zoe McLaren, a health policy professor at the University of Maryland. Exploring the mindset of physicians treating critically ill patients with COVID, she asks, "Is this actually working, or does it seem to be working because I want it to work and I feel powerless?"

Megan Coffee, an infectious disease doctor at NYU Langone Health, wonders if COVID's myriad clinical manifestations are a consequence of seeing many patients with the disease all at once.

"If you see enough cases of other diseases, you'll see unusual things," says Coffee, noting that, for those other diseases, such experience might take an entire career.

Elaborating on Coffee's perspective, Vinay Prasad, an oncologist at Oregon Health and Science University, worries COVID has acquired a clinical mystique, a perception the disease is so novel it calls for a radically different approach.

"Human beings are notorious for our desire to see patterns," Prasad says. "Put that in a situation of fear, uncertainty, and hype, and it's not surprising that there's almost a folk medicine emerging."

Perhaps Prasad had in mind POTUS, who suggested we drink or inject bleach, though the story of hydroxychloroquine is more illustrative. The severely flawed French study that caught POTUS's attention (not only did Didier Raoult, the lead French researcher, physically resemble Harold Bornstein, the President's former physician, their medical philosophies appear simpatico) abandoned quaint scientific notions such as control groups or randomized treatments. Raoult has responded to widespread criticism of his tactics by railing against the "dictatorship of the methodologists," as if the foundational precepts of clinical research are irrelevant.

POTUS promoted the drug, prompting a weeks-long orgy of Fox echolalia. Fake news, indeed.

The hysteria spread far and wide, infiltrating even the ranks of physicians, some of whom turned their backs on Hippocrates and wrote hydroxychloroquine prescriptions for themselves or their families. A good friend who runs Mayo's pharmacy told me of the sad situation in house—the numbers weren't large, but still—and I myself have refused an Rx request from a retired doc.

The magnitude of the COVID crisis has spawned similarly unprecedented research. Since the pandemic began, over 7,500 articles have been published, most online and not peer reviewed, ranging from letters to the editor decrying stigmatization of Asians to lead articles in the *New England Journal of Medicine*, the *Journal of the American Medical Association*, and the prominent British journal *Lancet*. The NIH's website is a great resource for collated research:

https://www.ncbi.nlm.nih.gov/research/coronavirus/ A less daunting alternative, volume-wise, comes from the NEJM: **http://www.jwatch. org/covid-19**

Remdesivir was initially trialed against Ebola in West Africa and found ineffective. Repurposed against COVID, results from two clinical trials made headlines last week.

Garnering the most attention was an NIH study whose results Dr. Fauci deemed "highly significant." For patients battling COVID, Fauci said, Remdesivir would be the new "standard of care."

It's worth exploring the details of the study to further illuminate the usually circumspect doctor's words. The NIH trial enrolled 1,063 patients infected with COVID, randomizing half to placebo and half to Remdesivir. The results, which are preliminary and unpublished, show the treatment group had a 31 percent faster time to recovery than those given placebo. (The "p value" of the study was < 0.001, which means the chance of the findings occurring by happenstance is less than one in a thousand, a statistically "highly significant" result.)

In the nuts and bolts section of the study, the aspect that's clinically relevant, Remdesivir-treated patients recovered, on average, in 11 days, while the mean days to recovery in the placebo group was 15. Mortality in the Remdesivir cohort was 8.0 percent, while the death rate in the placebo group was 11.6 percent, $p = 0.059$, a result not quite reaching statistical significance. (In a clinical trial, results are defined as "statistically significant" if the probability of the outcome occurring by chance is less than 5 percent.)

Statistical significance of a trial doesn't necessarily translate into *clinical* significance. The Helsinki Heart Study, published as a lead article in the *New England Journal of Medicine* in 1987, is a good example. In the trial, 4,000 middle-aged men without heart disease were randomized to receive, over five years, the lipid-lowering drug gemfibrozil or placebo. Results showed a 34% decrease in heart attack in the treatment group, $p < 0.02$.

I remember well "34 percent risk reduction" on buttons pinned onto expensive dresses worn by pretty Parke-Davis drug representatives who catered lunch when I was a resident doctor in Honolulu; Parke-Davis sponsored the research and manufactured gemfibrozil.

A deeper dive into the data is worthwhile. Over the five years of the trial, 41 of 1,000 men who received placebos had heart attacks, while the figure for the gemfibrozil group was 27; in 1,000 treated men, 41-27 = 14 heart attacks were prevented, so the relative risk reduction (RRR) ascribed to the drug was 34 percent. (14/41 = 0.34, or 34 percent.)

But a second look at the data tells a different story. Four point one percent of the placebo group had a heart attack, compared to 2.7 percent of those given gemfibrozil, meaning that merely 1.4 percent of the treated men benefitted from taking the drug. Analyzed yet another way, 71 men (the reciprocal of the absolute risk reduction (ARR) cited above, or 1/0.014 = 71) had to be treated for five years to prevent one heart attack. (Number needed to treat = NNT.)

At the time, even the prestigious *NEJM* didn't require ARRs or NNTs in its publication. Years later, researchers presented this data to doctors in varied formats. Would you prescribe a drug for five years that decreased the chance of a heart attack by 34 percent? If giving a drug to 71 patients for five years prevented one heart attack, would you prescribe it? Unsurprisingly, by a wide margin, the first scenario won out.

Now, gemfibrozil is used infrequently.

Chinese COVID research published in *The Lancet* the same day as the NIH study showed no statistically significant difference in time to clinical improvement or mortality in patients treated with Remdesivir compared with those given placebo. But just 237 patients were enrolled, half of what researchers had hoped (the epidemic in China was quickly controlled, and Chinese scientists couldn't locate enough patients to randomize) so the study wasn't adequately powered (more patients, more statistical power) to discern small treatment effects.

In 1987, Dr. Fauci led a team at the NIH that showed AZT was clinically helpful in AIDS, though it would be nearly a decade before this drug together with others was given as a cocktail that turned HIV into a chronic disease. The modest clinical success of Remdesivir against COVID, Fauci says, "is reminiscent of 34 years ago in 1986 when we were struggling for drugs for HIV."

WHITHER POLITICS?

May 7

How does a pandemic affect politics? In less than six months, God willing, we'll elect a new president. But compared to the same interval before past elections, going to the polls seems further away. Because we haven't been hearing as much about politics, it's receded from our minds. COVID has shoved everything else offstage, like our attention-craving POTUS. But social distancing—physical distancing is a more apt term—has drained the lifeblood from politics.

In a democracy, politics depends on social discourse. Citizens organize. They assemble in groups to support their candidate and knock on doors urging neighbors to do the same. Candidates hold town hall meetings, where they listen to voters' concerns. These interchanges both enlighten and enliven, energizing both citizens and candidates.

The virus has hollowed out our public space.

Normally, in late summer, we'd look forward to the Democratic and Republican conventions—thousands of loyalists waving flags, holding signs, and wearing weird hats—four days of boosterism for the man or woman chosen to pursue the highest office in the land. This summer, as always, the events will be televised, but without packed convention halls the spectacles may not earn the term, resembling Colbert from his home and without laughs from a television audience.

After Labor Day, rallies for the candidates typically swell in size. The night before the election, in front of huge crowds, Bruce Springsteen would headline for the Democrat while Lee Greenwood would croon *God Bless the U.S.A.* for the Republican. Six months from now—or 12, perhaps 18—the risk of COVID won't be less, so we'll miss out on, for worse or better, this political theater. Probably…

This should help Joe Biden, whose charisma deficit, compared to Barack Obama or Bernie Sanders or seemingly POTUS, for reasons beyond my ken (thousands applauding his misanthropy at his rallies may be the saddest facet of his tenure) puts him at a disadvantage. Anthony Scaramucci has said that eventually POTUS "turns on everyone and soon it will be you and then the entire country." Don Junior, has said that, other than golf, his dad just likes to win.

Will POTUS stage an October surprise? Besides winning at any cost, other considerations may fade from his mind like a mirage on the road. Might he flout the conventional wisdom of every sane American? Defy the advice of "experts" and stage massive rallies? The raised middle finger for which his base adores him, even as it imperils both them and their loved ones?

For a man who won't wear a mask in a mask-making facility, don't put it past him.

In November, will we mail in our votes? Or will we need to choose between voting and our health? (Fifty-two Wisconsinites who'd voted or worked the polls in the April 7 primary contracted COVID in the following two weeks, the majority in Milwaukee County.) It should go without saying that the founders didn't intend citizens to be forced to choose between staying alive and casting a vote.

Physical distancing restricts our politics, loosely defined, through other means. According to Hanna Arendt, a person's political power depends on the ability to work with her fellow citizens. "Loneliness is not solitude," Arendt wrote. "Solitude requires being alone whereas loneliness shows itself most sharply in the company of others," a sense I suspect many of us have experienced when immersed in a crowd. "What makes loneliness so unbearable," she continues, "is the loss of one's own self which can be realized in solitude but confirmed in its identity only by the trusting and trustworthy company of equals."

Thinkers throughout our history have commented on the relationship between isolation and democracy, and their perspectives are less straightforward than you might think. According to John Dewey, democracy "is not an alternative to other principles of associated life," but "the idea of community life itself."

Alexis de Tocqueville, on the other hand, worried that small "d" democrats in America—unlike aristocratic Europeans whose ancestral ties to their land made them "almost always closely involved with something outside of themselves"—would break this chain of inheritance, leaving "each man… forever thrown back on himself alone." This isolation, he thought, threatened to enclose a man "in the solitude of his own heart" and render America ripe for despotism.

De Tocqueville was writing in 1840, but we're at least as atomized now.

James Madison believed property owners would not readily "invade the rights of other citizens." Ensconced in their homes, this isolation, he thought, would provide a bulwark for representative government.

And there's a less theoretical aspect of politics.

For Betty Friedan, the "problem that has no name" was the isolation of the suburban housewife. Initially, "she was so ashamed to admit her dissatisfaction that she never knew how many women shared it." Then, on an April morning in 1959, having coffee with four other mothers, one mentioned, in a tone of quiet desperation, "the problem," and everyone knew that it wasn't her husband, her children, or her home. Four years later, Friedan published *The Feminine Mystique*.

Frederick Douglas was walking one day along the Baltimore wharf when he struck up a conversation with two Irish dockworkers. After hearing Douglas was enslaved for life, they suggested he flee north. Years later,

Douglas cited this random encounter as impetus for his escape. One of the tragedies of this pandemic is that such meetings, planned or chance, occur less often.

The virus has both exposed and exacerbated our society's inequities. Can they be remedied? Neither workers in meat-packing plants nor nurses in hospitals should have to labor in unsafe environments, but both groups face obstacles to collective bargaining. The people who process our food speak many languages. For many, if they don't work, they won't eat. Fear of deportation prevents advocacy. And nurses (shout out to our heroes during National Nurses' Week!) are loathe to leave their patients' bedsides to join picket lines.

But "essential" workers truly are so. From such a realization political power may emerge, though no one can believe that its exercise, by these people now, will be easy. But everyone should understand: on the essential among us, all of us depend.

AN OVAL OFFICE CHAT

May 8

"You're fired!" POTUS told COVID. The president and the pathogen were alone in the Oval Office.

The virus shook its head in disbelief. "You can't just fire me, POTUS," COVID said. "Just yesterday, according to the website Worldometer, I infected 29,531 of your subjects."

"Citizens," POTUS interjected. "It's not like I'm king or anything."

"Could have fooled me," COVID said.

"Well, um, thanks for the compliment."

"I didn't mean it as a compliment."

POTUS leaned forward, knitted his brow. "Do you know who you're talking to?"

COVID sat up straight, even straighter than it was, at risk of uncoiling its RNA. "Do *you*?"

POTUS's face went from orange to red. "You're fired, I said! Get the hell out!"

COVID shook its head. "I'm afraid you don't understand."

"What's there to understand? I fired you! You're out of my mind, so get out of sight!"

COVID chuckled. "I'm already invisible."

"The nerve of you!" POTUS swiped at COVID's chair, as if it were a fly to be squashed Obama-like. COVID feinted left, and POTUS missed.

"POTUS, please," COVID said. "Be reasonable."

POTUS sat back in his chair and sighed. The virus had seen this posture before as it lurked airborne during meetings of the White House Coronavirus Taskforce—an entire taskforce focused on it! the virus reflected gleefully— when Don Junior would barge in and utter something inane.

"I know you're busy," COVID said. "Thanks for taking the time." To convey anything to POTUS, anything at all, first you had to flatter him. The virus had seen Fauci and Birx take this tack, watched the doctors try to put a mask on their expressions, again and again, in response to POTUS's recalcitrant stupidity. Put a mask on. Now there's an idea, COVID thought. "That's a really nice tie you're wearing," the virus said. "The perfect color of red. And the length, well, I don't care what Comey says, it's just right."

"Thanks," POTUS said. "It was a gift from Marla." He inclined his head toward COVID conspiratorially. "Just don't tell Melania." POTUS gazed past COVID as if fantasizing of a faraway place. His look wasn't bliss—POTUS was too tortured for that; his mommy never loved him—but a nod in that direction, COVID thought. "The sex me and Marla had," POTUS continued pensively. "I mean, Melania's pretty and all, but compared to Marla, especially the last three years, she's a cube of ice."

"I can imagine," COVID said.

POTUS shot the virus a look.

"The sex with Marla, I meant," COVID said. "I can imagine *that*."

"Like hell you can!" POTUS said. "You're just a virus!"

COVID rolled its eyes. The coronavirus wanted to tell POTUS about all of the sex *it* had been having. Well, not sex exactly, but replicating, gazillions of times a day, creating COVID progeny at a rate of which POTUS could only dream. But it mustn't make POTUS feel inferior, COVID reflected, not if it wanted to get through to him.

Lately COVID, though not inclined to deep thoughts, had had some regrets. Sure, the virus wanted to live, live and reproduce, like all flora, fauna, and plague-causing microorganisms. But there'd been too much collateral damage, it had to admit, especially in the United States, where cases exceeded 1.3 million. Sometime this weekend, deaths COVID had caused in America—deaths it had contributed to; some people died from blood clots, or strokes, or heart attacks, or secondary bacterial infections; the virus refused to fasten its seatbelt and go on a guilt trip—would exceed 80,000. The stats weren't close: the world leader was leading the world.

Across the globe, people pitied the United States, whose woeful leadership had caused needless suffering. The virus felt bad for Americans but had no sympathy for the president, who was too King Lear-ish to notice, much less care about, what anyone thought.

"Look," COVID said. "I know you're worried about the economy."

"Of course I am!" POTUS said. "We've got to get people back to work!"

"I understand," said COVID, trying to forge a bond. "The unemployment rate is at 14.7 percent, the worst it's been in 80 years, and in the last seven weeks, the economy has shed 33 million jobs."

POTUS sighed. "Don't remind me."

"It's not like it's your fault," COVID said. Of course a lot of it *was* his fault—if POTUS had taken COVID seriously, if he'd believed in test, trace, and quarantine, if he'd mandated masks and encouraged social distancing, America wouldn't be in this economic pickle—but saying so wouldn't help its cause.

"I know, I know," POTUS said.

"But here's the thing," COVID said. "You can deal with both at the same time."

"Huh?" POTUS asked. "Both?"

COVID nodded. "If you focus on me it'll help the economy." The virus had thought of saying "get rid of" instead of "focus on" but feared sufficiently for its survival the way things were. Bad enough to ask POTUS to focus on it—not that he was much of a focuser—which wasn't exactly in the virus's interest.

"You know what?" POTUS asked. "For the last two months, three months, whatever, all I've been doing is focusing on you!"

"Understood," COVID said. "And by the way, thanks for resurrecting my task force."

"You're welcome. I had no idea how popular the task force was until actually three days ago when I started talking about winding down."

COVID nodded; the syntax was jumbled, as usual, but the virus got POTUS's point. It thought the task force should stay in place, perhaps, because COVID was still maiming and killing, not because the task force was popular, but provoking POTUS wasn't smart. Not if the virus were to accomplish its mission.

The night before, COVID had hardly slept. History, the virus worried, would consider it a serial killer. When COVID made the leap from a bat to a pangolin to a shopper in a Wuhan wet market, joining the ranks of Gein and Gacy and Dahmer wasn't what it had in mind. Time to fall on its sword, COVID thought. Stop this American carnage! "Sir," it said. "If we could get back to the economy."

POTUS nodded enthusiastically. "It's the economy, stupid! Even Bill Clinton knew that!"

"Correct," COVID said. "If you do beaucoup tests, find out exactly where I'm living, and if you isolate all of those people, and track down all of their contacts, and then quarantine them, pretty soon..."

POTUS held out his hands as if to push COVID away. "Aren't you listening! I said it's the economy!" POTUS took a breath, scooted back in his chair. "Sorry," he said. "And that's a word I never say. But I didn't mean to go off on you."

"No problem," COVID said. "Your job is stressful."

POTUS shook his head scornfully. "The lamestream media never gives me a break. *The Washington Post* especially. Jesus, I hate Jeff Bezos. Bastard's even richer than me"—POTUS leaned forward, cupped his hand to his mouth, and whispered, "I'm not as rich as people think. Why do ya' think I won't release my tax returns?" His voice flipped back to bombast, per routine. "I'm a smart guy! But wanna know what really bothers me about Bezos?"

"What?"

"His girlfriend's even hotter than Melania."

"That sucks," COVID said. In truth, it didn't get it, this fetishism for the female form. Procreation for the virus was sufficiently satisfying all by itself; well, with a smidge of human help.

"Bezos," POTUS sneered. "The fake news *Washington Post* says in my first three years of being president, I lied over 16,000 times." POTUS paused. "I haven't counted, but between you and me, they're probably right. But I'm gonna throw Bezos and everyone else the best curveball they've ever seen."

"Whatcha gonna say?" COVID asked.

"For once, tell the truth."

"Really? Care to elaborate?"

"What d'ya' think I've been doin' my whole life? Back in February, I said you'd go away. And a week ago I doubled down, like I do, because I'm right." POTUS tapped on his noggin. "It's all up here," he said. "The truth is, you'll go down to zero. The virus will. In the end."

"Please, Mr. President," COVID said. "It's not, I'm not, that simple!"

"Nonsense!" POTUS said. "You're disappearing! Right now! Get the hell out!"

"O.K." COVID had tried. Tonight, conscience clear, it would sleep soundly. The virus extended its hand—no elbow bumps for this numbskull—which POTUS shook.

COVID walked out. Where could it go? Who would it find? The frustration, the total waste of its time, made the virus want to reproduce.

VACCINES TO
THE RESCUE!

May 9

The race is on! The competition for a COVID vaccine makes the rivalry between Salk and Sabin (Albert Sabin was one of the first in a long line of immigrant physician-scientists to help make American medical research the best in the world) resemble a chess match between two geezers in a park. Over 100 pharmaceutical companies or groups of researchers are working toward the goal. Operation Warp Speed, POTUS calls it.

Finding and manufacturing a vaccine is an urgent priority, arguably the most important endeavor in the history of science. To the winner or winners, glory and profits will accrue. It's worthy of a world-wide Manhattan Project.

All the more tragic that POTUS, as a political ploy, has defunded the WHO, which is well placed to coordinate such an effort. Billions of vaccine doses need to be distributed across the globe, for humanitarian reasons and because, as with smallpox and polio, residual pockets of COVID anywhere threaten us all.

The U.S. government has partnered with Johnson and Johnson in a $1 billion-plus effort to make a vaccine, but a phase one clinical trial—which merely monitors toxicity in volunteers—isn't slated to start until September.

Massachusetts-based Moderna has received close to half a billion government dollars to fund trials of its vaccine candidate. Phase 1 was completed in March, and the biotech company is now proceeding with phase 2, which will monitor, in 600 vaccine recipients, safety and production of antibody that Moderna hopes will confer COVID immunity. If phase 2 goes as smoothly, the company hopes to start phase 3 by early summer, enrolling thousands of volunteers to be observed for side effects and immune response to the vaccine.

Moderna has made a so-called mRNA (messenger RNA) vaccine, which instructs cells to produce the spike proteins that give the coronavirus its name. COVID's distinctive spike protein is an example of an antigen, a protein found on the surface of viruses and bacteria, which the human body recognizes as foreign and the immune system responds to by making antibodies.

If the FDA finds it safe and effective, Moderna has partnered with Swiss drugmaker Lonza to manufacture up to a billion doses of vaccine. Pfizer, too, is working on an mRNA vaccine.

These mRNA vaccines may not work. The technology is new, and no such vaccines have been approved by the FDA against any microorganism, though an mRNA vaccine against the chikungunya virus, which is endemic in India, sub-Saharan Africa, Haiti, and parts of South America, has generated protective antibody in early trials.

On the other hand, mRNA technology, compared to other modes of making vaccines, is more readily scalable to the industrial production needed to make billions of vaccine doses, and there's no molecular biological reason why it shouldn't work.

Last month researchers at Beijing-based Sinovac Biotech reported that, for the first time, a COVID vaccine protected an animal from subsequent infection. The Chinese scientists made their vaccine the old fashioned way, chemically inactivating a version of the virus and inoculating eight rhesus macaques with two different doses of this vaccine. Three weeks later, by sticking a tube down the (anesthetized) monkey's windpipes, the scientists introduced COVID into their lungs. The highest-dosed monkeys showed no sign of COVID, the monkeys given the lower dose had a "viral blip" but didn't get sick, while a control group of four unvaccinated macaques developed severe pneumonia and had evidence of viral RNA throughout their bodies. Three days ago, their research was published in the prestigious journal *Science*. Phase 2 trials will start soon.

Sinovac is an experienced vaccine maker that has successfully marketed inactivated vaccines for hand, foot, and mouth disease; hepatitis A and B; and bird flu. But the technology is more difficult to scale; the company says at most it could produce 100 million doses.

They needn't worry about Gary Bauer (or others who share his political-religious biases), the "Christian" activist who's said that "when a vaccine is developed, the drug company making it better not manufacture it in China, no sane American would take it." Methinks he protests too much, unless Mr. Bauer prefers to meet his maker sooner than he might have planned.

In the race for a vaccine, researchers at Oxford's Jenner Institute had a head start. Based on safety data compiled on a vaccine for MERS, one of two other serious illnesses caused by a coronavirus (the third is SARS), they convinced British regulators to proceed with a phase 2 COVID study involving 6,000 people, as England's epidemic rages on.

Their technology genetically modifies a harmless virus to make a COVID look-alike, which stimulates an immune response without causing disease. As with Sinovac, the Oxford researchers inoculated six rhesus macaques with their vaccine and then exposed them to COVID. In the following month, the macaques have maintained their health.

The Oxford Group expects results from its phase 2 trial in mid-June, but the preliminary findings were sufficiently promising for British pharmaceutical giant AstraZeneca to partner with them to ramp up vaccine production. The Oxford researchers don't expect to conclude the all-important phase 3 trial, the final step before regulatory approval, until September—if they're green lit for it because of a successful phase 2—but the Serum Institute of India, the world's largest vaccine maker, plans to produce 40 million doses of the vaccine before then. Taking this step before a drug is found safe and effective, and prior to regulatory approval being obtained, is unprecedented, a risk for which the Indian company should be praised.

Operation Warp Speed, if perhaps not in the United States.

But there is hope.

A GOOD MASK
IS HARD TO WEAR

May 10

Forget abortion, or gay rights, or Merry Christmas, or even hydroxychloroquine. The latest front in the culture wars is face coverings.

It's a front in the war against COVID, too, of course, though to say we're waging war against the virus isn't true. Yes, the battle rages, but the fight is one sided. The enemy is relentless, lethal, employing stealth to the max, its invisibility almost a metaphor. Though everyone wants the virus gone, 40 percent of the country acts as if it already is. You can't expect to win a war if you fail to as much as acknowledge the presence of the enemy.

In Flint, Mich., a Family Dollar security guard was shot and killed for enforcing Michigan's law requiring masks for anyone entering a public space. Also in Michigan, for the same reason, a customer at a Dollar Tree wiped his face on an employee's shirt.

Americans are famously libertarian, and there's a longstanding tension between the public's health and individual freedom. Depending on the issue, our laws come down on one side or the other. New Hampshire is the only state in the union without a mandatory seat belt law; if you're injured in a car accident, advocates for such laws would argue, state taxpayers may have to pay for your care.

It's no surprise that Harley-Davidson has adopted New Hampshire's Live-Free-or-Die motto. In Western Europe, motorcycles are more common than in America. And while it's uncommon to see a helmetless rider in Europe, an American on a Harley wearing a helmet is a rarity.

Thirty-seven states require testing and disclosure of radon levels during real estate transactions; 13 don't.

"A well regulated militia, being necessary to the security of a Free state, the right of the people to keep and bear arms, shall not be infringed." Books have been written about the interpretation of this ambiguous amendment. But before *District of Columbia v. Heller,* in 2008, a 5-to-4 Supreme Court ruling dividing conservatives and liberals on the court and across the nation—a decision made possible by a generation of judicial scholarship paid for by the Federalist Society and the N.R.A.—declaring D.C.'s handgun ban unconstitutional, public protection arguments had a chance.

At the 2016 New Yorker Festival, after a panel discussion on armed citizens, I approached Jonathan Mossberg, currently CEO of Kalashnikov USA. The public health literature, I said, suggests that a gun in the home is more likely to be used by a member of the household against another family member or him or herself than against an intruder. He cut me off by saying, "You're making a paternalistic argument." I thought for a moment, nodded, and walked away.

Indeed I was. Mossberg seemed to have conceded my point. His family might *not* be safer with guns in his house. But in his opinion, *he* should make the decision and not the government.

Perhaps second-hand smoke is most analogous to the (sadly contentious) issue of masks in America. Currently, 35 states ban smoking in bars, restaurants and workplaces—a list that grows each year—and more than 22,000 municipalities covering 82 percent of the population have similar laws. In an enclosed space, one person's smoking affects another's health, with bartenders and wait staff in smoke-filled bars at highest risk.

Whereas secondhand smoke can worsen asthma, precipitate a heart attack, or cause lung cancer, the mere act of breathing or talking can spread COVID. Can and often does: a substantial percentage of transmission is from infected people who display no symptoms.

Wearing a mask can prevent this occurrence. At Mayo, everyone wears a mask. In the exam room, my mask protects my patient and her mask protects me. Ditto Menard's. But at Festival Foods, well-run otherwise, clients and staff make up their own minds. Late afternoons, few shoppers or employees wear masks. (We'll see if this changes now that cumulative cases in Eau Claire County have nearly doubled in a week, from 28 to 54, maybe because the Minneapolis metro, during that interval, has become a COVID hotspot.) Early mornings at Festival, however, time set aside for older shoppers, almost all customers wear face coverings.

Some states have mask mandates. Michigan, as mentioned, which has left some protestors hot in the uncovered face. Maryland, Pennsylvania, New Jersey, Connecticut, and Illinois residents must cover their faces in essential businesses. New York requires it when social distancing isn't possible; e.g. on the subway. Hawaii requires masks for anyone venturing outside of their home, enforced by a fine of as much as $5,000 or a jail sentence of up to a year.

In Stillwater, Ok., a very red state, officials received so much verbal abuse over a mandatory mask law that it was dropped within hours. In response, Norman McNickle, the city manager, said, "It is unfortunate and distressing that those who refuse and threaten violence are so self-absorbed as to not follow what is a simple show of respect and kindness to others."

Compared to Asia, we're not used to wearing masks. The CDC's guidance has flip-flopped from "don't wear a mask unless you're a health care worker" to "wear one in a public space." And POTUS, per his divisive and anti-science wont, has seized on the mask issue, manufacturing controversy with which to stoke his base. Wearing a mask would make him appear weak! By not wearing one, he's holding up his middle finger not just to COVID but to the conventional wisdom of wimpy intellectuals like Nancy Pelosi and

Mayo Clinic CEO Gianrico Farrugia, who insist on wearing one because it's smart and it's kind—I can't be sure I don't have COVID, so I'm doing my part to prevent the virus from infecting you.

But it's a hassle to wear a mask. They're uncomfortable. We don't look good with them on. Ya-da-ya-da-ya-da. Masks aren't a habit, and habits take time to turn into the same. And we don't want to be perceived as weaklings. We descended from Neanderthals, you know, when if confronted by a saber-toothed tiger, well, it's an evolutionary biological kind of thing.

I myself have experienced this. When I wear a mask in a convenience store, which I always do, a blue collar guy might walk by and give me a look. Not scorn, exactly, but fairly close. I'm overreacting, he's thinking. Worse, I scare easily. And guess what? Part of me is actually afraid, just a bit. Not of an altercation but of being seen as a wuss.

Pitiable POTUS, discouraging his rank and file from wearing masks, makes other nations pity us. We won't wear masks. And we won't isolate cases of COVID away from their families. And we won't trace contacts of these cases and do the same. And so we beat on, our boat against the current, borne ceaselessly into the past, destined to be buffeted by wave upon wave of COVID, breaking over our prow, threatening to sink our ship.

Shout out to mothers! Thank you, Mother, for keeping me on the straight and narrow—or trying to.

YOU THINK YOU'VE
GOT IT TOUGH?

May 11

It's not possible to fly into Haiti commercially. All airlines have suspended service. No doctors, nurses, or relief workers can obtain passage there.

It's not as if Haiti doesn't need help. Grinding poverty, political unrest, dysfunctional government, an abundance of endemic disease: HIV, cholera, tuberculosis, Dengue fever, chikungunya, malaria, and now, COVID.

At St. Luc's Hospital—improvised from shipping containers to treat victims of the 2010 earthquake—in Port-au-Prince, they're doing their best. Now, with the invasion of a novel microorganism, added space is an urgent priority.

With the arrival of the first official case, on March 16, Father Rick Frechette and his team renovated the cholera wing of the hospital, raising the roof to increase air flow and decrease heat.

I can testify to how helpful these adaptations might be. Most of St. Luc's lacks air conditioning, and temperatures in May soar into the upper 90s, accompanied by drenching humidity. Fans circulate the hot air, which by late morning exceeds 97F, the temperature of human skin, at which time one steers clear of them. Seeing patients with my Haitian colleagues, who wore shirts and lab coats, their brows didn't glisten, while my scrubs were perpetually soaked. I rehydrated with pint after pint of water at the hospital and bottled Coke made from local sugar cane—liquid manna from heaven—at the end of the day.

In a country without reliable sources of clean water, conserving it and sodium, instead of sweating them out, may have helped Haitians survive, a benefit perhaps offset by the prevalence of severe hypertension in the country, where it's common to see 20 and 30-somethings presenting with strokes.

This initial renovation of St. Luc's—rewiring electricity for lights and fans followed raising the roof—opened 40 beds for treating COVID patients. Cases increased, prayer followed, funds came in, and new shelters were created for families to help them care for their sick.

Yet more cases, still more prayer, additional funding. Families were moved to a different area and the vacated space, now equipped with power lines and running water, was further renovated with toilets and showers to open 40 new beds.

Father Rick is a man of great faith, his needs often met, well, as if by acts of God. One night 10 years ago, he was trying to salvage a large bell, toppled by the earthquake from a church's steeple. He prayed for a backhoe (in Haiti, heavy equipment is rare) and soon one rolled around the corner; to hear the priest tell the story, embellished by his grins and laughter, is close to divine.

The outpatient clinic has also been repurposed to treat patients with COVID, for whom the hospital now has ninety beds. They're considering other sites as necessary, including the Villa Francesca Guest House at which I was booked two short months ago, before COVID and a surge of kidnappings halted, for the time being, my research on peripartum cardiomyopathy (severe heart failure that occurs in women in the last trimester of pregnancy or in the first few months after giving birth, a disease of which Haiti has the world's highest incidence) a collaborative endeavor between Mayo and UW-Eau Claire.

Haiti has only 182 confirmed COVID cases and just 15 documented deaths, but surveillance is poor; the country has administered only 1,300 tests. Father Rick reports "disastrous delays" receiving test results.

At St. Luc's, patients suspected to have COVID range in age from 17 to 92. Of 200 such patients, "about" 85 were hospitalized and "about" 13 died. Of these 85, "about" 20 had the virus officially. Of the 13 deaths, three were confirmed COVID positive.

Such are the difficulties of caring for the sick in a resource-poor country, to say nothing of inadequate PPE that has caused two St. Luc's doctors to take ill.

The government advises people to stay indoors, which isn't possible if you're hungry. In sprawling Port-au-Prince, population 3 million, 850,000 residents need more to eat. Chaotic scenes of the government distributing parcels of food to the neediest seem likely to spread the virus.

Political unrest, poverty, and an inadequate health care infrastructure—the country of 11 million has only sixty ventilators and just one doctor for every 15,000 residents—create a "perfect storm," according to the UN, which warns of a looming "humanitarian catastrophe."

In Kano, Nigeria, 400 kilometers north of Jos, where I once spent a week, the gravediggers know something is up. One told the BBC death had not come to the city so quickly in 60 years, when a cholera epidemic had raged. Obituaries in local newspapers display the names of many thought to have died from the virus. On a recent Saturday, two professors, a newspaper columnist, the former editor of a paper, and the mother of a Nigerian movie star were among COVID's probable casualties. But nobody knows, because none of them were tested.

According to Worldometer, Nigeria's COVID caseload totals 4,400, with 143 deaths. But the most populous nation in Africa has administered only 24,000 tests. A week ago, in response to hardship (starving citizens) the Nigerian government ended a lockdown that had been in place for more than a month. Non-essential businesses have reopened, even in Lagos, population

21 million, though masks are required in any public space. In this realm, one of POTUS's "shithole" countries is outdoing us.

Prime Minister Narendra Modi locked down India on March 24, when the country had 519 documented COVID cases. (As can be inferred, the actual number was much higher.) India has a large system of trains, which abruptly stopped, precipitating a humanitarian crisis for migrant workers desperate to get home; many walked hundreds of miles. Tomorrow, the trains resume running. Otherwise, the lockdown continues.

Officially, the country now has recorded 70,000 COVID cases and 2300 deaths, with new cases and deaths recently averaging a respective 3,500 and 100 each day. Though the country of 1.3 billion has done only 1.6 million tests, hospitals haven't reported surges. Yet. But food insecurity plagues 255 million Indians, who the lockdown has further impoverished. Under intense pressure, Modi intends to start easing restrictions next week.

With Haiti, Nigeria, and India, with every nation on earth, we'll watch what happens and hope for the best.

FALSEHOOD FLIES

May 12

Falsehood flies, and the Truth comes limping after it, wrote Jonathan Swift.

Swift's surmise was confirmed in an ambitious study of social media published two years ago in the journal *Science*. The scope was massive. MIT researchers analyzed every major contested news story—some 126,000 in all—tweeted by 3 million users over a span of more than a decade. Their conclusion? By every metric, falsehood comes out on top. Fake news and false rumors reach more people and penetrate deeper and faster into the social network than does the truth.

"False information outperforms true information," said lead researcher Soroush Vosoughi, a data scientist. "And that is not just because of bots. It might have something to do with human nature."

I'd agree.

"We must redesign our information system in the 21st century," wrote 16 political scientists and legal scholars in an accompanying essay, urging more research "to reduce the spread of fake news and to address the underlying pathologies it has revealed." They called for a novel "news ecosystem… that values the truth." It's still a pipe dream.

A false study is more likely to go viral than a true story, the researchers found, reaching 1500 people six times faster. False news outperforms the truth in every category—business, science and technology, entertainment—but political fake news flies the fastest.

On average, compared to true stories, tweeters prefer to share lies. Even when the scientists controlled for differences between accounts that spread rumors, including the number of followers or if the account's owner was verified, lies were 70 percent more likely than verities to be disseminated.

The two lead scientists endured a two-day lockdown after the April 15, 2013, Boston Marathon bombings during which wild conspiracy theories held sway on social media. When they reunited on campus, they decided to research what they'd just been through.

On social media, why do lies succeed? The MIT team settled on two hypotheses: novelty and emotion. False tweets are often notably different from tweets appearing in a user's account over the prior two months, and lies more frequently elicit surprise or disgust.

"False information online is often really novel and frequently negative," said Brendan Nyhan, a professor of government at Dartmouth. "We're attentive to novel threats and especially attentive to negative threats."

"The key takeaway is really that content that *arouses strong emotions* spreads faster, more deeply"—more re-tweets by different users—"and more broadly on Twitter," wrote Rebekah Tromble, a political scientist at Leiden University in the Netherlands.

A lie repeated often enough becomes accepted truth. The quote has been attributed to Lenin and Joseph Goebbels, Hitler's propaganda minister.

On April 30, POTUS was asked if he'd seen evidence that COVID had emerged from a Wuhan lab. "Yes, I have," he said, nodding gravely. "Yes, I have." POTUS pivoted to the WHO, seamlessly weaving the agency into his latest conspiracy theory. "I think the World Health Organization should be ashamed of themselves because they are like the public relations agency for China," he said, a quick 180 from earlier statements praising the country for their pandemic response. "They shouldn't be making excuses when people make horrible mistakes, especially mistakes that are causing hundreds of thousands of people around the world to die." Three days later, Minister of Disinformation Mike Pompeo went on ABC to announce that there was "enormous evidence" that COVID had originated in a Wuhan lab.

Both men refused to provide any evidence, because evidence doesn't exist. The theory has been widely debunked by scientists, who note that nature is far more adept at creating SARS and COVID and bird flu and countless other (thankfully) benign viruses than any researchers, however malevolent their intent, could hope to be.

Not only is truth irrelevant but also facts can blunt propaganda's effectiveness, as POTUS and Minister Pompeo understand. "Hillary Clinton may be the most corrupt person ever to seek the presidency," said POTUS, to great effect. "Lock her up!"

Last night, I watched a bootleg copy of *Plandemic*, 30 minutes of slick propaganda worthy of Leni Riefenstahl, which, in a matter of days, had been watched by millions of viewers before being removed by YouTube, Facebook, Twitter, and Vimeo for "violating community guidelines" and in order to "halt the spread of misinformation."

The film focuses on Judy Mikovits, a discredited former researcher. Narrator and filmmaker Mikki Willis opens by saying, "Now, as the fate of nations hangs in the balance, Dr. Mikovits is naming names of those behind the plague of corruption"—including Anthony Fauci, against whom she has a special animus and who she links without evidence to the Wuhan lab—"that places all human life in danger."

"If we don't stop this now, we can not only forget our republic and our freedom, we can forget humanity; because we'll be killed by this agenda," Mikovits says.

Among the clip's many untruths is a humdinger: wearing a mask weakens your immune system, increasing your susceptibility to COVID. For your health, don't mask up! The "documentary" recycles conservative tropes: evil experts connected to a deep-state-like mechanism of surveillance and control, grievance, and a sense of persecution. The clip even extols the benefits of hydroxychloroquine. Mikovits' book based on the same malarkey is a top seller on Amazon.

I've often wondered about the affinity of self-described Christians (four of five evangelicals supported POTUS in 2016, a figure that is little changed) for a man whose personal behavior and political agenda is antithetical to the message of the Gospels. But on further reflection, the love affair is easily explained. POTUS's "Christian" base believes in him with the same religious devotion with which they believe in Christ's resurrection. Surprising—shocking, really—to rise from the dead. Memorably so. Besides, when you believe in someone, truly love him or her, no amount of evidence will change your mind.

Believers believe; skeptics are skeptical.

When my love swears that she is made of truth, I do believe her, though I know she lies, Shakespeare wrote.

I saw a patient yesterday, a retired elementary school teacher, a woman in her 80s. She hadn't been a reliable Republican, not until 2016, when something she can't describe about POTUS captured her fancy and made her vote for him; she'd said this two years ago when I'd asked her opinion about the president. She didn't inquire about mine. POTUS supporters, in my experience, never do. When you believe in someone…

Her husband died nine years ago.

"I don't care if I get the virus," she told me yesterday.

"Why would you say that?" I asked non-confrontationally.

"If I get it and die, I'll see my husband."

Fourteen years ago, a study explored the possible benefit of intercessory prayer for patients having heart bypass surgery. In 2020, it seems quaint that such a proposition would be put to scientific test, a vestige of a bygone era, like laws against interracial (or gay) marriage, which now seem ridiculous.

The study, funded by the late billionaire investor and evangelical Christian John Templeton, was prospective and double-blind, the gold standard for a clinical trial. Patients were told they might or might not receive prayer. Group 1 was prayed for—per personal routine but including "for a successful surgery with a quick, healthy recovery and no complications." Group 2 went without. No difference in complications or mortality was observed.

It's doubtful that Sir John saw the irony of his position, hoping for a positive result, which would have demonstrated the efficacy of distant prayer. Such an outcome would have proven, one might surmise, the existence of God. Though if God were real, he or she might frown on the endeavor, consider it hubris. Prove I exist? How dare you! That's *my* bailiwick!

But what if the trial results had been reversed? If researchers had "proven" the existence of God?

Perhaps there'd be fewer true believers.

AMERICAN
EXCEPTIONALISM

May 13

"A lockdown is a means and not an end," said Firass Abiad, who oversees COVID efforts at Lebanon's main government hospital in Beirut. "It's a means either to allow you to regain control or put measures in place to control coronavirus when it comes back. When we eased the lockdown, we knew there would be an increase in the number of cases."

Yesterday, responding to an uptick in COVID cases, Lebanon reimposed restrictions almost exactly two weeks after easing them up. In the small country (population 6.8 million), there were 36 new cases on May 10, up from a baseline beneath five.

Last week South Korea rescinded a go-ahead for bars and clubs after scores of new cases were linked to such venues in Seoul. In the nation of 52 million, in the last four days, new cases total 122. In the prior two weeks, daily numbers were less than 10.

"It's not over until it's over," said South Korean President Moon Jae-in. "We must never lower our guard regarding epidemic prevention."

Germany has seen localized outbreaks and has warned that restrictions might need to be reinstated.

"We always have to be aware that we are still at the beginning of the pandemic," Angela Merkel said. "And there's still a long way to go in dealing with this virus in front of us."

Six days ago Germany's COVID reproductive number, or R0—the number of persons an infected person goes on to infect—(if the value is < 1, an epidemic is waning while > 1 means the opposite) had dropped to 0.65, and Merkel said Germany could "afford a bit of courage" while warning that "we have to watch that this thing does not slip out of our hands."

But over the weekend, officials at the Robert Koch Institute (RKI), the German equivalent of the CDC, said R0 had again climbed above one. RKI noted "a degree of uncertainty" with R0 estimates, but the increase "makes it necessary to observe the development very closely over the coming days."

Merkel, who has a PhD in quantum chemistry and was a research scientist before entering politics, works closely with the RKI on infection control policy, which the federal government implements in cooperation with the states. If a German county has more than 50 new cases per 100,000 residents, lockdown measures will be reintroduced. Over the weekend, several counties surpassed that threshold.

The data seem to have been a statistical blip. Over the last four days, new cases in Germany again number less than 700, where they've been since the start of the month, except for May 6, 7, and 8, when the average approached 1,200.

Germany, population 83 million, has registered 174,000 cases and 7,792 deaths since the pandemic's start. In the U.S., four times as large, cases exceed 1 million and the death toll is approaching 90,000.

China, too, is enforcing new restrictions following a total of 16 (in a country of 1.3 billion) newly confirmed cases. The city of Shulan, which borders Russia and North Korea, has been put under lockdown after 11 new cases were diagnosed. And in Wuhan, five new cases were confirmed, again about two weeks after the city started emerging from its singularly effective but draconian lockdown.

"Stay alert and step up personal protection against the virus," said Mi Feng, spokesman for China's National Health Commission.

In the United States, new cases in the last week averaged 25,000, a slight decrease from the weeks before, when the mean had been ~ 30,000; there's been some progress, but we're far from bending our curve. Compared to China, South Korea, and Germany, our public health response to COVID—at best—has been tepid.

Lebanon has also responded more robustly to the virus than has the United States. The nation's first case, on Feb. 21, was in a plane passenger arriving from Iran, which a day earlier had reported *its* first case. Schools and universities were shuttered eight days later, and Lebanon locked down March 15. The economic fallout in a country already dealing with its worst-ever economic crisis was a factor in a phased reopening at the end of last month.

In America, 40 states are in the process of reopening their economies. None have satisfied all White House Coronavirus Task Force criteria to safely do so, according to frequent CNN contributor Dr. Leana Wen, who was interviewed yesterday by the BBC. Shortcomings include a lack of decreasing cases in the most recent two weeks; suboptimal testing capacity for patients with COVID symptoms; inadequate ability to trace contacts of infected cases (Dr. Wen suggests the U.S. needs an additional 166,000 workers for this purpose); and inadequate surveillance testing to detect pockets of symptomless infection, which would serve as an early warning system for a regional outbreak. A chagrined Dr. Wen added that our ability to quarantine contacts was even worse.

Yesterday in remote testimony before the Senate HELP committee, Dr. Fauci was asked about the consequences of premature opening. "My concern is that we will start to see little outbreaks," he said. "The consequences could be really serious."

When asked about Fauci's comments today, POTUS said, "It's not an acceptable answer. We're opening our country. People want it open."

Willful blindness, just like his flock.

If the above is a view from 35,000 feet, Atul Gawande, in today's *New Yorker*, offers suggestions for businesses to safely reopen based on hospitals' experience doing the same.

Gawande suggests combination therapy, "like a drug cocktail" that consists of hygiene measures, screening, distancing, masks, and last but not least, creating a caring work atmosphere. Hand washing has been documented to decrease the spread of respiratory pathogens. Employees should self-screen and stay home if they're sick. Distancing and masks, no more need be said.

The fifth component—a culture of caring—may be most challenging. Humans, Gawande says, "tend to focus on two desires: keep me safe and leave me alone." Employees need to embrace "the desire to keep others safe, not just myself." If you've got a sore throat, stay home. If a co-worker's mask has slipped below his nose, gently remind him to pull it up, and expect your colleagues to request this of you. My mask protects you, and your mask protects me. One for all, all for one.

It's the culture of the operating room, he says, "wanting, among other things, never to be the one to make someone else sick."

A lockdown is "a means either to allow you to regain control or put measures in place to control coronavirus when it comes back," said Lebanon's Dr. Abiad. The control we've regained is meager, and our measures to control the virus upon its inevitable return are inadequate. In less than two months, we seem to be capitulating, giving up the will to wage war against a virus that Angela Merkel tells us has just begun.

In their scientific stoicism and the solidarity she's inspired, the Germans emulate their leader. In our lack of discipline, we resemble ours. Some may say we deserve him, but I disagree.

Americans are better than POTUS. We just need someone to remind us, a leader to show us the way.

SAVE THE ECONOMY!
PRINT MONEY!

May 14

The headline from the Bureau of Labor Statistics is 14.7 percent unemployment, but the BLS indicated the rate would actually be close to 20 percent if the survey had accounted for gig workers and temporary layoffs. Neither did the number include people who couldn't file claims because of overwhelmed state unemployment offices.

Whatever the actual figure, the magnitude of jobs lost and the speed with which it has happened are unprecedented in U.S. history. Three million more Americans filed for unemployment benefits this past week; total COVID-related job losses stand at a staggering 36.5 million.

True, the underlying economy had been healthy and growing pre-virus, a solid foundation for an eventual recovery, but an ongoing risk of contagion, cash-strapped consumers, and businesses shutting their doors permanently are strong headwinds against a brisk economic rebound. Billionaire hedge fund owner and former George Soros protégé Stan Druckenmiller says the prospect of a v-shaped recovery is a "fantasy." Druckenmiller, who's 66, says the risk-reward calculus for stocks is the worst he's seen in his career.

But the stock market is not the economy, as Paul Krugman and others remind us, and it's in the real economy where people are struggling. The virus may be an equal opportunity pathogen, but our fellow citizens already facing precarity suffer the most.

Before the virus hit, half of Americans lived paycheck to paycheck. Since the dawn of the pandemic, 40 percent of families earning less than $40,000 annually report at least one household member is out of a job.

Consumer prices dropped by 0.8 percent last month, seasonally adjusted, the biggest drop since 2008. And while falling prices might be good for household budgets, they're low because shoppers don't have money to spend. When prices fall because consumers aren't spending, manufacturers can't turn a profit. Workers are laid off, meaning there are less dollars yet to be spent, triggering a vicious cycle.

To combat this potential economic calamity, Congress has passed four separate pieces of legislation costing a cumulative $2.4 trillion. The largest is the $2 trillion CARES Act, which paid $1,200 to low and middle-income adults. Federal unemployment benefits of $600 a week will be guaranteed through the end of July. A payroll protection plan (PPP) provided $349 billion in forgivable loans to small businesses, as long as the money went for salaries, utilities, and rent. When funds quickly ran out, an additional $380 billion was allocated. In addition, $250 billion for hospitals and COVID testing was approved.

"The scope and speed of this downturn are without modern precedent, significantly worse than any recession since the second world war," Federal Reserve chair Jerome Powell said yesterday. "While the economic response has been both timely and appropriately large, it may not be the final chapter, given that the path ahead is both highly uncertain and subject to significant downside risks. Additional fiscal support could be costly but worth it if it helps avoid long-term economic damage and leaves us with a stronger recovery."

House Democrats have proposed such a stimulus in an additional $3 trillion bill designed to support state governments, which face a cash crunch because of sharply diminished tax revenue; to ramp up testing; and to extend unemployment benefits through January.

What's Nancy Pelosi up to? Wouldn't it be better, politically, to let POTUS and his loyalists reap the pitiful harvest they've sowed? Does she want to force Republicans to vote against her plan? Hoist them upon their proverbial petard? Or is she a stateswoman pursuing the public interest?

Extending unemployment benefits seems necessary because of how we, compared to some European countries, have gone about fiscal stimulus. Denmark has paid companies to retain employees, compensating workers up to 90 percent of wages. As a result, Denmark's unemployment rate is 10 percent lower than ours. Kurzarbeit—a German state-funded program dating to the post-WWII era created to help companies adjust to difficult times without resorting to mass layoffs—reimburses workers 60 percent of lost income, a little more if the worker has children at home.

Uniquely in the United States, health insurance is tied to employment, so a layoff means you're uninsured, too. Sure, under COBRA, you can buy your company's coverage at the going rate, or purchase it on the open market. But losing your job in America—if you're lucky enough to have one with health insurance—is a double whammy: lost income and incoming health care bills.

You might wonder how the current fiscal stimulus stacks up against the government response during the financial crisis and the recession it caused a decade earlier. Three pieces of legislation, in 2008, 2009, and 2010 (the latter memorably named TARP), provided a total of $1.4 trillion ($1.67 trillion in today's dollars) in economic stimulus.

The Fed, too, is pulling out all stops. Quantitative easing (QE) during the financial crisis, from Nov., 2008, through Oct., 2014, saw the Fed purchase bank debt, mortgage-backed securities, and Treasury Bills to push money back into the economy. (Theoretically, at least: of $4 trillion in increased money supply through QE's nearly six-year duration, banks kept $2.7 trillion in cash reserves rather than lend it per the Fed's intent.)

When the Federal Reserve purchases securities, it adds to its balance sheet, which eventually, they tell me, it's supposed to pay off.

Did you know the Fed can draw down its IOUs merely by not renewing a T-bill upon maturity? Me, neither. For this chemistry major, the Fed's machinations are as magical as Angela Merkel's mastery of quantum chemistry.

At the peak of the Fed's monetary interventions, in June, 2010, its balance sheet was plus $2.1 trillion. How do the Fed's actions then compare to now?

By the end of 2020, the Fed is expected to buy $3.5 trillion in securities, increasing its balance sheet by the same amount. And earlier this week, for the first time in history, the Fed bought a new class of assets: corporate bonds included in exchange-traded funds. Merely the program's announcement had the desired effect. In late April, Boeing, without help from the Fed, successfully raised $25 billion by selling bonds; the Fed, bond investors concluded, has the bond market's back.

The Fed has suggested it might, in the future, purchase *individual* corporate bonds, perhaps even junk bonds. Purchasing bonds raises their prices—more dollars chasing the same supply of goods—which keeps the bond's interest rate low, making it cheaper for the issuing company to borrow cash. Capiche?

There are limits to what fiscal and monetary policy can do to rescue economies, which ultimately sink or swim because of the goods and services that people will buy. In the era of COVID, for that to occur, workers and consumers must feel safe.

It's happening here at Mayo. Patients are returning; internists like me are examining them in our offices; surgeons are operating. This morning alone, I saw 10 patients! It's likely the environment won't be perfectly safe. Some of us may fall sick.

But the risk is acceptable, and incumbent on us to take; we want to care for our patients in the manner doctors and nurses do. We're trying our best to adhere to Dr. Gawande's culture of the operating room, to prevent anyone from getting sick.

When consumers and workers at businesses throughout the country feel like we do at Mayo, the U.S. will be well on its way.

I'd doubted demand for medical services would return this quickly. Humility is important, dealing with COVID and in general. I was wrong, as I've been before and will be again.

LEGISLATING
FROM THE BENCH

May 15

A year ago, in wondrous pre-COVID New York City, Monica and I, two months before marrying in a magical ceremony in front of cherished family and friends, attended a Broadway play. I'd read about "What the Constitution Means to Me" in a *New Yorker* article three months earlier and at once was intrigued.

In high school, playwright Heidi Schreck, who starred in the production, competed in American Legion Oratorical Contests, giving speeches on the U.S. Constitution for prize money. During her high school career, Schreck did well enough to pay for college; as a senior, she raked in $4,000 as the national runner-up.

"I really did believe there was no greater democracy on the planet, and that this document was the most genius piece of political writing that had ever been created," Schreck recalled.

Her views have changed. As epilogue to the play, Schreck and teenage Rosdely Ciprian debated the topic, Should We Abolish the U.S. Constitution?

The production, a Pulitzer Prize finalist, was by turns hilarious, poignant, and thought provoking. The topic is women's rights, including abortion—Schreck herself had one in her early twenties—and the jurisprudence of Roe v. Wade. Schreck entertainingly explicates the Ninth Amendment—"The enumeration in the Constitution, of certain rights, shall not be construed to deny or disparage others retained by the people"—about which Antonin Scalia once commented, "If my life depended on it, I couldn't tell you what the Ninth Amendment was." If he'd lived to see Schreck's play, a light might have flickered on for him.

"This means that just because a certain right is not explicitly written in the Constitution, it doesn't mean you don't have that right. The fact is there was no possible way for the framers to put down every single right we have—the right to brush your teeth, sure, you've got it, but how long do we want this document to be? Here's an example: When I was a little girl, I had an imaginary friend named Reba McEntire. She was not related to the singer. Just because the Constitution does not proclaim the having of an imaginary friend as a right, does not mean I can be thrown in jail for being friends with Reba McEntire."

In 1965's *Griswold v. Connecticut*, the Supreme Court, in a 7-2 ruling, found that a married couple, instead of the state of Connecticut, could decide whether or not they used birth control. Writing for the majority, William Douglas said this right was located within the "penumbras" and "emanations" of other Constitutional protections. In a concurring opinion, Justice Arthur Goldberg invoked the Ninth Amendment.

Onstage in New York, the audience was treated to an audio recording of oral arguments before the court in which Douglas and the Griswold's attorney were heard to cough nervously; sex was such a delicate topic; contraception, likened to feminine hygiene, was the province of women alone; the theater set was a Legion hall hung with portraits of august Legionnaires, all white and male, a mirror of the court.

Thus did the Ninth Amendment afford a right to privacy that guaranteed abortion rights, or so Norma McCorvey and her lawyers believed, as have millions of women and men before and after the 1973 Supreme Court decision, arguably the most controversial in our nation's history.

In college I read Harry Blackmun's majority opinion. At the time, I was a political science major, considering a degree in law. I found the decision fascinating, though I disagreed with its conclusion. To me, abortion was simply wrong.

As a college freshman, I would have described myself as a conservative, as were my parents (we've long since evolved) but abortion had never come up. So I was taken aback when, home from college, my mother took me to task for presuming *I* could decide what was obviously a woman's choice.

Like Schreck's views on the Constitution, mine have changed on abortion. I've come to believe the ruling on Roe was a compromise: until a fetus is viable, an abortion is legal. After that, a state can intervene. In that sense—where to draw the line—the decision found middle ground.

Decades ago, my first wife and I went to a Christmas dinner sponsored by a local nursing home. We arrived late, and just one table had open seats. We joined an older couple, the four of us at a table for eight.

Somehow, after wine and hors d'oeuvres, conversation drifted to abortion. The man was a family doc in an outlying town, and his very Catholic wife was strongly "pro-life." She described Catholic teaching on the rhythm method, how Catholics view barrier contraception as interfering with the will of God, His wherewithal to create a human life.

"That's beautiful," I said. "It only becomes ugly when you try to ram it down somebody's throat."

The evening ended amicably, and I learned something.

Regarding abortion, most of us can agree that abortion in early pregnancy isn't "murder"—the vast majority of Americans wouldn't send a woman to prison for taking a "morning-after" pill to prevent a just-fertilized egg from implanting in the uterus—while also believing that late-trimester abortion on demand is abhorrent. Somewhere in between, government can and should intervene.

Anti-abortion activists accuse the court, in Roe, of judicial activism. Legislating from the bench.

They have a point. While the 1967 *Loving v Virginia* decision banning state anti-miscegenation laws has been relegated to a bygone era, people of good will continue to stand on both sides of an abortion divide caused by a court ruling merely six years later.

Years ago, in *The Atlantic*, Jeffrey Goldberg argued that abandoning Roe might serve liberals well. Repealing it, after all, won't criminalize abortion. That would be up to the states, where legislators would have voters to answer to. Goldberg's point was two-fold: only the reddest states in the Deep South would limit abortion, and conservatives would be deprived of a wedge issue with which to get out the vote.

Without Roe, Hillary Clinton would be president.

Liberals don't have a monopoly on judicial activism. In 2010, a conservative court not only ruled Citizens United could screen a film critical of Hillary Clinton shortly before the 2008 Democratic primary in violation of the 2002 campaign finance reform law, it equated speech with campaign contributions, thereby affording the latter expansive First Amendment rights. And who can forget *Bush v. Gore*, where the Supreme Court, by the slimmest of margins, told Florida to stop counting votes?

The latest example of conservative judicial activism? The Wisconsin Supreme Court, which knows better than an elected governor how best to balance the Badger State's economy and its health. In a 4-3 decision, the court struck down Governor Tony Evers' safer-at-home initiative, permitting all states businesses, including bars and restaurants, to reopen at once, and marking the first time any statewide order of its kind has been knocked down by a court of last resort.

"This decision will undoubtedly go down as one of the most blatant examples of judicial activism in this court's history," Justice Rebecca Dallet wrote in dissent. "And it will be Wisconsinites who pay the price."

HEARTS AND MINDS

May 16

Yesterday was difficult. I walked into an exam room where my patient sat next to his wife. He was wearing a MAGA hat.

A problem I'd never faced. In fact, to my recollection, I'd never talked with anyone wearing one. Now, that conversation could not be postponed.

In January, on a plane bound for Hawaii with my wife, a man beneath a MAGA hat sat on the aisle. Walking past him, I fought the urge to slap it off his head. It's an inclination I've struggled with before, seeing MAGA on somebody's head, thinking whoever was wearing it (always a white man) was a moron or evil or maybe both.

It pains me to admit this. I've talked to scores of POTUS supporters, most of them patients, and know they're good folks. They love their families, get up in the morning and go to work, and desire the future for our country they consider best.

Still. MAGA is a trigger, as it is for POTUS's boosters. The slogan was political genius—perhaps the only intelligence of which POTUS is capable—proudly brandishing a raised middle finger at the coastal elites, political correctness, abortion-rights activists, the *New York Times*, CNN, the academy, or wonkiness of any stripe.

POTUS's name on a hat or t-shirt provokes me, too, but not as much. Perhaps I subconsciously see MAGA people at POTUS rallies, when they were a thing, cheering every disgusting and defamatory comment he spews. There *does* seem something wrong with them.

Though maybe I compartmentalize. My patients, good people, wouldn't be found in such a crowd. Or was it that my patients were good people—even the ones decked out in MAGA merchandise—if only I got to know them?

Whichever. MAGA hats still piss me off, as if the wearer has to advertise his allegiance to a narcissistic and ignorant bully, blaring, That's my guy!

But the day wasn't hard because of MAGA man. In fact, he was a pleasure to deal with.

While a nurse was putting Mr. MAGA into an exam room, I was next door, talking to an elderly patient who'd presented for an annual physical. I left him to change into his gown and walked into my office, where I was given sad news.

A few minutes later, I returned to my elderly patient and sleep-walked through his exam. Then I went next door and saw the red hat. A slight blessing of my distressing news was that MAGA faded into the background.

My patient was in his 70s. I've taken care of him for less than a year. He has diabetes, and kidney and heart disease. He and his wife looked blue collar, lower middle class. Both are heavy, she's heavier, clad in a t-shirt.

I'm ashamed to admit I don't know what he did for a living. Farmer? Janitor? Computer programmer? Probably not, but you never know. Maybe he was still working. Frequently, farmers never stop. Get to know someone in a MAGA hat, I'm thinking now, as I write.

He was feeling better than the last time I'd seen him and pleased about that. I tried to focus on his blood sugars, suggested an increase in his dose of insulin.

I'd first met him two years earlier, when he was establishing care with another doctor and came in with an acute problem when that physician was unavailable.

Monsieur Le Maire, I'd called him, a play on my patient's given name, referring to Hugo's protagonist, the title taken by Jean Valjean after he worked his way up from poverty to become mayor of Montreuil-sur-Mer. My patient had heard of *Les Miserables*, or so it seemed, but Monsieur Le Maire was news to him. But he smiled as I explained the connection, perhaps forging one between the two of us, maybe part of the reason he later switched to my care.

Our political opponents aren't our enemies. If we listen more than we talk, we can forge new relationships. Regarding politics, such connections may be our best chance to win hearts and change minds.

HOW TO BE A RACIST

July 22

A dozen miles southwest of Ashland, Wis., in the far northern part of the state, is the town of Benoit. The unincorporated village sits along a county road, where it elbows two miles north to U.S. 2, after having traveled a like distance west from U.S. 63. Besides the Benoit Cheese Haus, featuring curds made from 19-year-old cheddar, there's no reason to visit. Certainly my wife and I, on a recent vacation, wouldn't have passed through en route to Bayfield, a charming Lake Superior community; a detour diverted us.

Bayfield County, along with Ashland and Douglas Counties to the east and west, are islands of political blue amidst a sea of Republican red north of U.S. 8, a landscape of lake and forest sprinkled with taverns, dotted with hardscrabble farms, and graced by an occasional church.

No blue in Benoit, not a Biden sign in sight. Instead, POTUS signs sprouted like spring dandelions from nearly every lawn we drove by. There seemed to be more placards hailing the 45th president than the hamlet had residents. It made me wonder, taking in the magnitude of Benoit's devotion, if POTUS himself had once stopped there, purchasing and gorging on mounds of Wisconsin curds.

Because whatever prosperity in America POTUS might take credit for, and he takes credit for it all, any suggestion of affluence, besides the cheese house with its burgundy shutters and spotless white concrete-block edifice, appeared to have eluded Benoit, where paint peeled off ramshackle homes.

Why is the town in love with 45? Doubtful Benoit's citizens have reaped much benefit from the CARES Act, especially the $454 billion set aside for large corporations through a lending program run by the Fed; using the moolah as collateral, the Fed has nearly $4 trillion with which to buy bonds, driving their prices high enough for investors to purchase stocks instead, a phenomenon applauded by Steven Mnuchin and his Wall Street pals. Besides a $1,200 stimulus check and soon-to-expire $600/week unemployment payments, what has POTUS, in conjunction with Congress, done for Benoit?

POTUS love pursued us north to the Bayfield Inn, where young men in ball caps blaring MAGA thronged the rooftop bar like so many thorns on a rose. The scene in the harbor, sailboats on the great and placid lake, Apostle Islands in the background, was lovely otherwise. Nor could we escape MAGA in a t-shirt shop, where the owner, face uncovered, kept watch over his POTUS merchandise.

Apostle Islands Booksellers had a different vibe, the window lined with books on racial justice, no MAGA-clad men inside. I was reminded of a radio interview with Garrison Keillor a couple years back. When asked how he felt about his country, Keillor responded, "I love America. I love (dramatic pause) its geography. The wide expanse of prairie, the majestic mountains, the shining sea. It's Americans I don't always appreciate. You see, I hang around people who go to libraries, who read books."

I picked up a novella entitled *The Meursault Investigation* wherein Algerian author Kamel Daoud gives both a name and narrative to the unnamed Arab murdered by the eponymous protagonist in *The Stranger*, by Albert Camus. Workers had masks on; shoppers, too, were required to wear them. Howl, an outdoor clothing store, and the Bayfield Artists' Guild Gallery, also had mask mandates. Weird to know a proprietor's politics by whether or not masks are required. Sad that wearing a mask has become political, when, according to researchers at the University of Washington, 95% compliance with public mask-wearing could, by the November election, save 40,000 American lives.

The day after we returned from our trip, I sat reading Ibram X. Kendi's National Book Award-winning *Stamped From The Beginning, The Definitive History of Racist Ideas in America*. The title is from a speech on the Senate floor by Jefferson Davis opposing a bill funding black education in Washington, D.C. "This government was not founded by negroes nor for negroes," he said. The "inequality of the white and black races" was "stamped from the beginning."

Mr. President, can you see why it's objectionable to fly the Confederate flag? Why statues of men like Davis, rather than "preserving our history," are symbols of white supremacy? And Mitch McConnell, POTUS's chief enabler, why would you say it's "nonsense that we need to airbrush the capitol and scrub out everybody from years ago who had any connection to slavery?"

I glanced up from my book and gazed out the window, where the wind whipped cirrus clouds, shearing pieces from their peripheries, honeycombed fragments, whirling unhurriedly, forming and then melting away, resembling the CT scans of COVID-infected lungs.

In a recent Fox News interview with Chris Wallace, POTUS said, "I'll then make a speech. It'll be a great speech. And some young guy starts writing, Vice President Biden said this, this, this. He didn't say it. Joe doesn't know he's alive, OK? He doesn't know he's alive." About COVID, "I will be right eventually. You know I said, It's going to disappear. I'll say it again."

When asked about removing the names of Confederate generals from U.S. military bases, POTUS replied, "We're going to name it after the Rev Al Sharpton? What are you going to name it, Chris? Tell me what you're going to name it!" He added, "So there's a whole thing here. We won two world wars, two world wars, beautiful world wars that were vicious and horrible. And we won them out of Fort Bragg. We won out of all of these forts that now they want to throw those names away."

Given such comments, and his ineptitude with the virus (COVID has been a political gift to any world leader with a modicum of empathy and competence) I keep checking 538, Nate Silver's website, waiting for the president's approval rating to dip below 40 percent, but it won't budge.

I don't get it. Most everyone I know can't fathom how POTUS has more than single-digit support. But the people I know go to bookstores, at the window displays of which his followers avert their gaze.

During the 1980 presidential campaign, Rosalyn Carter said Ronald Reagan made people comfortable with their prejudice, which helped explain his popularity. Reagan's racist dog whistles—starting his campaign in Philadelphia, Miss., close to where three civil rights workers were murdered 16 years earlier, with a speech extolling states' rights—have become POTUS's megaphone.

In the two months I've been away from my blog, my patients have made some interesting comments. "I don't understand these folks," said a retired male professor, referring to demonstrators in the wake of George Floyd's murder. "They burn down their stores and then complain about having no place to shop." He pointed to his head. "Something's wrong with their thinkers."

Another retired man, an engineer with a master's degree: "I guess I don't really have time anymore to listen to other views. Then again, I just watch Fox." When I brought up the NFL, wondering if they'd have a season, he said, "Not if they play a black national anthem. Fans will boycott the games." Just yesterday, a retired woman, also college educated, said she watches Fox because they cover the news more thoroughly than the competition and then let the viewers decide. POTUS's Fourth of July Mount Rushmore talk, she told me, was "the best speech I've ever heard."

Excerpts: "Our nation is witnessing a merciless campaign to wipe out our history, defame our heroes, erase our values, and indoctrinate our children. Angry mobs are trying to tear down statues of our founders, deface our most sacred memorials, and unleash a wave of violent crime in our cities."

"One of their political weapons is cancel culture, driving people from their jobs, shaming dissenters, and demanding total submission from anyone who disagrees. This is the very definition of totalitarianism."

Another patient is an American success story. After running away from an abusive father at age 13 and surviving for a time on the streets, he eventually became manager of a local creamery. He's grown disenchanted with South Texas, where he and his wife have wintered since he retired. "You know," he said, "those Mexicans are taking over Texas. They're dirty people. Really, they don't bathe. There's no telling what germs they could bring with them. The virus. They could give us the virus. And those blacks in Minneapolis," he added, sadly shaking his head. "Looting their stores, destroying their neighborhoods."

MLK: "A riot is the language of the unheard."

"I guess I'm a racist," said another patient with a laugh. "I mean, these blacks complain about not having any jobs, but they won't go to college. If they'd just go to college, they'd get jobs, you know?"

How much of POTUS's appeal to his supporters in Benoit and to his supporters everywhere is because he makes them comfortable with their prejudice? To what extent is Fox News popular for the same rationale?

Why do white people need to feel superior? How can we whites—each of us—search for and eradicate the lingering bias in our hearts and minds?

HEALING AMERICA

July 26

In the United States, for the four days ending July 24, daily deaths from COVID exceeded 1,100, a figure not seen since early June. Far and away, in cases per capita, we lead the developed world.

In deaths per person, we're also closing in on global leadership.

Probably, before the November election, we'll be number one. Why? Because, unlike almost every other western nation, we've failed to control the virus. Since June 24, the seven-day average of new cases has more than doubled, from 31,402 to 66,100 a month later. (We're testing more people, which leads to more cases, but the percentage of positive tests has also increased.)

More worrisome, nearly 60,000 Americans are currently hospitalized with COVID, roughly the same as on April 15, when a record 59,940 COVID patients were in the hospital. According to the CDC, in the four weeks starting April 11, daily deaths averaged 2,180. Can we expect, in the month to come, a doubling of daily deaths?

Hopefully not. Drug treatments such as Remdesivir and dexamethasone have helped, as has placing patients, if they can tolerate it, in the prone instead of supine position, to better aerate the anterior lung, which, compared to the posterior aspect, COVID is less likely to destroy; the practice of proning delivers precious oxygen where it best can be put to use. More young people, because they're less likely to wear masks or social distance, are becoming infected and hospitalized; relative youth confers a survival advantage. Then again, according to Worldometer, more than 19,000 Americans are now critically ill, several thousand more than the average of April's pandemic peak.

A year ago, at a friend's birthday party, I met a young man, an Army Ranger, buff from hours in the gym, whose t-shirt proclaimed, "I believe in American exceptionalism." I didn't confront him—it was a party—but I suspect this sort of exceptionalism wasn't exactly what he had in mind.

Any president with an iota of competence or compassion could have mitigated this calamity.

Not POTUS. In the two months I disappeared from cyberspace, he's held a rally in Tulsa (I thought he might try to stage big events in the fall as an October surprise, but never dreamed he'd endanger his adoring hordes, and anyone with whom they'd interact, by such megalomaniacal narcissism this soon in the campaign); spoken in front of more unmasked supporters on the Fourth of July; withdrawn from the WHO; had his Justice Department file an amicus brief against the ACA's constitutionality, jeopardizing health care for 23 million Americans; and criticized Anthony Fauci, since 1984 the nation's top infectious disease doctor, forcing Fauci to obtain extra security because of threats against him and his family by right-wing goons, causing the good doctor to wonder out loud, "Is this the United States of America?"

Only this week has POTUS bowed to reality, or paid heed to his poor standing in the polls, canceling his Jacksonville re-coronation show—give him a coronavirus crown, which would be nicely symbolic; who would as much as consider a packed convention in the hottest of the nation's virus hot spots?) and at long last encouraging mask wearing, even troubling himself to Donald one.

But though POTUS has been integral to America's woeful COVID response, he hasn't been sufficient. Give me your tired, your poor, your huddled masses yearning to breathe free, the wretched refuse of your teeming shore? Hardly. One nation, indivisible, with liberty and justice for all? The reality doesn't come close to matching the rhetoric.

COVID has shone a bright light on America's inequities. The poor—essential workers making minimum wage—don't have the luxury of working from home, where they'd be safe from the virus. The huddled masses of mostly black and brown Americans living beneath one roof—aunts and uncles, cousins and grandparents—can't social distance. Refugees—wretched refuse from faraway lands—lose their lives in meat-processing plants so we can eat pulled-pork sandwiches.

"No scientific doubt exists that, mostly, circumstances outside health care nurture or impair health," says Don Berwick, former administrator of the Center for Medicare and Medicaid Services and professor of pediatrics and health care policy at Harvard Medical School. "Except for a few clinical preventive services," he notes, "most hospitals and physician offices are repair shops, trying to correct damage from suboptimal social determinants of health," which he describes as conditions of birth and early childhood; education; work; the social circumstances of elders; community resilience, including adequate transportation, housing, and safety; and perhaps most importantly, a sense of fairness that sufficiently redistributes wealth and income to give everyone a measure of security.

Though we spend $3.6 trillion dollars a year on health care, an average of $11,000 for every man, woman, and child (50 percent more than any other nation), Berwick suggests a good share of this money is being misspent. In the U.S., 40 million people are hungry, almost 600,000 are homeless, and 2.3 million are incarcerated and have minimal health services, of whom 70 percent have mental health and/or substance abuse issues.

Deep and pervasive structural racism continues to deprive black and brown people of opportunity while shearing years off their life expectancies. From midtown Manhattan to the South Bronx, life expectancy declines by 10 years—six months for every minute on the subway. From Chicago's Loop to the city's west side, the loss of life expectancy in years is a full 16. From the affluent centers of these cities to their disadvantaged communities of color, conditions and their consequences change drastically.

What if we invested in actual human well-being, Berwick wonders? What if we raised taxes to improve social determinants of health, or shifted money from an "overbuilt, high-priced, wasteful, and frankly confiscatory system of hospitals and specialty care" to the cause? I agree with Dr. Berwick that this won't happen unless we embrace what he calls the *moral* determinants of health—attack racism and other social determinants while creating a sense of solidarity allowing all Americans to "depend on each other to help secure the basic circumstances of healthy lives, no less than they depend legitimately on each other to secure the nation's defense."

How to do it?

Ratify the following UN agreements on basic human rights, which the U.S., alone among western countries, hasn't signed: the International Covenant on Economic, Social and Cultural Rights, the Convention on the Elimination of All Forms of Discrimination Against Women, the Convention on the Rights of the Child, the Protection of the Rights of All Migrant Workers and Members of Their Families, and the Convention on the Rights of Persons with Disabilities. Companies and countries write mission statements in order to keep their eyes on the proverbial prize, placing goals front and center; I myself was unaware these treaties existed, much less that we'd failed to sign them, until I read Berwick's recent essay in *JAMA*.

Make health care a human right, he continues. Again we stand alone among developed countries as 30 million Americans are uninsured, causing more than 10,000 unnecessary deaths each year. In response to the U.S. having the highest income inequality among G-7 nations, the billionaire Steven Mnuchin recently said, "I don't believe the redistribution of wealth is the right solution. I believe the right solution is to create equality of opportunity." There's no equality of opportunity if you die because you don't have health insurance.

Achieve radical reform of the criminal justice system, which incarcerates black and brown people five to seven times as often as it does whites.

Pass compassionate and comprehensive immigration reform legislation.

End hunger and homelessness.

Stop the attack on science by crucial government agencies.

Resist voter suppression tactics.

Abolish the Electoral College, permitting everyone's vote to count the same.

"Healers are called to heal," Berwick says. "When the fabric of communities upon which health depends is torn, then healers are called to mend it."

Citizens, too, are called to act, to do their patriotic duty, to help America fulfill the promise of its founders: *E Pluribus Unum*.

On Nov. 3, our choice will be stark. One man wants to deepen division, exacerbate inequity, while the other will bind up the nation's wounds and work to restore the health of the body politic.

Please, remember to vote.

Addendum: Somewhat ironically, COVID hospitalizations in the U.S. peaked at 132,500 on January 6, the day of the capitol insurrection.

Second addendum: A Stanford University study of 18 Trump rallies found them responsible for more than 30,000 documented cases of COVID and over 700 deaths.

WE MUST
DISENTHRALL OURSELVES

July 29

In August 1619, 12 years after the English settled in Jamestown, they purchased 25 enslaved Africans from English pirates, who'd stolen them from English slave traders, who in turn had abducted them from modern Angola. In the future United States, it marked the start of 250 years of slavery. In all, 12 million blacks were forcibly taken from Africa to be shackled and shipped across the Atlantic. Two million failed to survive the journey. Only 400,000 made it to the U.S., while the others disembarked on Caribbean or South American shores.

Four hundred years later, the *New York Times* published the 1619 Project, the brainchild of 2017 MacArthur Fellow Nikole Hannah-Jones, winner of this year's Pulitzer Prize for commentary. The goal? Reframe American history by considering what it would mean to regard 1619 as the year of our nation's birth.

Tom Cotton is vehemently opposed. The Arkansas senator has introduced a bill entitled the Saving American History Act of 2020 to "prohibit the use of federal funds to teach the 1619 Project by K-12 schools or school districts."

POTUS agrees with his wannabe. "I just look at—I look at school," he said. "I watch, I read, look at the stuff. Now they want to change—1492,

Columbus discovered America. You know, we grew up, you grew up, we all did, that's what we learned. Now they want to make it the 1619 project. Where did that come from? What does it represent? I don't even know."

He won't listen, but Ms. Hannah-Jones could inform him.

In 1945, her father was born in Mississippi into a family of share-croppers. A few years later, her paternal grandmother packed up her few belongings and her three young children and boarded a train, which took them to Waterloo, Iowa, fleeing the state that led the nation in lynchings and the county that set the standard for the state, where black men were hunted down and hung for "crimes" such as entering a room occupied by a white woman, accidentally bumping into a white girl on the street, or trying to start a sharecroppers' union.

In 1962, at 17, hoping to escape poverty, her father joined the army—of all ethnicities, percentage-wise, blacks have been and continue to be most likely to serve our country in the military. Another hope: by serving his country, his country might at long last treat him as an American.

It wasn't to be. He was discharged under murky circumstances and held down a series of menial jobs for the rest of his life. Her father, like every-one in her family, believed in hard work, but like everyone in her family, he couldn't get ahead.

From the corner lot of Nikole Hannah-Jones' childhood home, which divided the black from the white side of the Iowa town that had been redlined by the federal government, her father flew an American flag.

She didn't get it. In school, she learned through "cultural osmosis" that the flag wasn't really theirs; blacks had contributed little to make America great. How could her father, seeing how his country had abused, and kept abusing, black people, fly his flag with pride? His patriotism embarrassed her. The flag rippling in the breeze—though the paint on their house was perennially chipped, the flag was promptly replaced as soon as it started to tatter—to her seemed a symbol of his degradation.

But her father, she later discovered, had been right to fly his flag. She came to understand how it belonged to black Americans. Perhaps, fighting to realize their country's ideals, which preceded successful struggles against discrimination based on gender, nationality, ability, and sexual orientation and identity, the flag belonged more to them than to anyone else.

Blacks had cleared the land in the American southeast. They'd taught the colonists to grow rice. They'd picked the cotton that at the height of slavery accounted for two-thirds of the world's supply. They'd lugged the railroad ties permitting cotton to travel to northern textile mills that fueled the Industrial Revolution. They'd built the plantations of George Washington, Thomas Jefferson, and James Madison, which to this day attract visitors eager to gaze upon these memorials to American ideals: all men are created equal, endowed by their creator with certain inalienable rights, among them life, liberty, and the pursuit of happiness. Their unfree hands had laid the foundations for the White House and the Capitol and even placed the Statue of Freedom atop the latter's dome.

Black slaves made whites in the North and South very rich; at one point a Rhode Island slave trader was the second richest man in America. Profits from their stolen labor helped pay off America's war debt and finance the founding of prestigious universities, which blacks, defined as subhuman and incapable of higher learning, could not attend.

Blacks were sold at auction like cattle. They could be murdered or raped with impunity. They couldn't legally marry, or go to school. Their children belonged to their owner, who could sell them at will. They could be, and often were, worked to death.

This violence against blacks continues, exemplified by George Floyd's murder.

We must disenthrall ourselves, Lincoln said, and then we shall save our country.

State-sanctioned violence against ethnic minorities is part and parcel of American history. Andrew Jackson, whose portrait POTUS hung in the

Oval Office, is remembered for the Indian Removal Act, which forced Native Americans west of the Mississippi. In the process, he ignored a Supreme Court decision written by Chief Justice John Marshall in *Cherokee Nation v. Georgia*. "If courts were permitted to indulge their sympathies, a case better calculated to excite them can scarcely be imagined," Marshall wrote. He created for the Cherokees a new legal entity, "domestic dependent nations," "in which the laws of Georgia can have no force, and which the citizens of Georgia have no right to enter," and summed up his opinion by saying, "The Acts of Georgia are repugnant to the Constitution, laws, and treaties of the United States."

In response, Jackson is rumored to have said, "John Marshall has made his decision. Not let him enforce it." On the forced march of 800 miles known now as the Trail of Tears, one in four Cherokees died.

The American Indian Wars dragged on for most of the 19th century. Native American casualties numbered in the tens of thousands.

During a skirmish on April 25, 1846, 11 American soldiers were killed by Mexican troops. It wasn't clear who fired first, or if the 11 had been standing on American or Mexican soil. But Congress, in a Tonkin-like ploy, gave President James Polk authorization for the war that he'd sought. Two years later, when this war of aggression came to an end, the top half of Mexico was the lower third of the United States. The nearly 100,000 Mexicans who chose to remain in what was now U.S. territory faced worsening racial animosity.

Violence is integral to the American character, celebrated in the novels of Cormac McCarthy, the movies of Quentin Tarantino, and the NFL, where predominantly black athletes are exhibited at an annual combine, like slaves on an auction block, chosen by coaches hired by wealthy white owners, players who face, after the conclusion of their professional careers, a one-in-four chance of developing chronic traumatic encephalopathy.

We kill each other with guns far more often than in any other western country, actual American carnage, of which blacks suffer more than their share. The world's most powerful military—we spend more on it than the next ten countries combined—all too frequently fights wars of choice to justify its existence.

So it goes. No surprise that COVID infects and kills more ethnic minorities, as a percentage, than it does whites.

That Andrew Jackson's portrait still hangs in the Oval Office shines light on POTUS's cavalier attitude toward this suffering, his total lack of concern.

PLAGUES, NOW AND THEN

August 2

"Masks don't work," said my patient, a retired RN. "There's no scientific evidence."

I countered that scientific evidence did, indeed, confirm their effectiveness.

"Not with these kinds of masks," she said, nodding at my surgical mask while touching hers, sewn of cloth.

"My mask protects you, and your mask protects me," I said. "Other than maybe Menard's," I added, an attempt at levity, "this is the safest place in town." In truth, the clinic probably is *the* safest place in town, because every patient is screened for fever and COVID symptoms before they walk in the door. In the last two months, when the clinic has been open for business and mask wearing has been universal, I'm unaware of *any* transmission of the virus between patients and staff.

"How about hydroxychloroquine for prophylaxis?" she asked.

Her husband, whom I'd seen the week before, was the Fox devotee who'd said fans would boycott the NFL if, before games, the black national anthem was played along with the Star Spangled Banner.

"Believe Fauci, not Fox," I said.

"I'd like to see the *real* statistics on deaths from H1NI," said a second patient, a retired investment banker. "The media, don't get me started. They're blowing up problems—big time—from this coronavirus."

I nodded. Pick your battles. And with patients, don't go to war. Besides, I was running behind, a good reason not to Google the data then and there; only later did I learn there were 60.8 million cases, 274,304 hospitalizations, and 12,469 U.S. deaths during the 2009-2010 H1N1 pandemic, according to the CDC, which says the corresponding figures for COVID, through today, are 4.5 million cases and 151,000 deaths.

How many are currently hospitalized? Who knows? The administration has told hospitals not to share data with the CDC and report it instead to the DHHS. According to NPR, a contract to collate these stats was awarded under shadowy circumstances. Simultaneously changing the company doing the counting and the agency for which it counts is concerning, to say the least.

Most experts think deaths from COVID are underestimated because they're not so labeled unless a death certificate explicitly states. Cases are undercounted still more dramatically, according to recent data from the CDC. Studies looking at viral antibodies have shown that since the pandemic began, the prevalence of infection, symptomatic or not, is anywhere from two to 13 times higher—depending on where the tests had been run—than earlier reports had implied. Unsurprisingly, at 23, New York City has the highest percentage of positive serological tests.

"We've never done this before," said another retired RN, shaking her head in dismay. "What if we kept daily tallies of cases and deaths from the flu?"

Again I nodded. In the last decade, 2017-2018 was the deadliest influenza season, with an estimated 61,000 U.S. fatalities, while in 2011-2012, the least deadly season, 12,000 are believed to have died.

But what if my patients, inaccurate though their supposed facts are, have a point? *Are* we overreacting to COVID? How much caution is appropriate, and how much is excessive?

Researchers at the University of Washington, whose modeling of COVID mortality is followed closely, now estimate that when we go to the polls on November 3, the virus will be killing 1200 Americans each day. By the end of the year, it's reasonable to presume 150,000 more Americans will die, raising our death toll to 300,000 or maybe more.

Many of those deaths will have been preventable.

Former presidential candidate and POTUS pal Herman Cain, who died from COVID on July 30, may have been one of them. He'd attended POTUS's June 20 Tulsa rally, where he'd posted pictures of himself and his friends in which none wore a mask. On June 29, he tested positive for the virus and was hospitalized two days later. He may have paid for his loyalty to POTUS's sociopathy with his life; only a sociopath would knowingly place friends and supporters squarely in harm's way for the sole purpose of feeding his ego.

Though some may say Cain got his comeuppance for giving COVID his middle finger, any preventable death is a tragedy. Still, for the sake of my give-me-liberty-or-give-me-death conservative friends—give-me-liberty-AND-give-me-death?—I'll share some perspective.

Compared to the influenza pandemic of 1918-1919, COVID won't be as deadly. At a time when the U.S. population was 100 million, 675,000 Americans died. Irrespective of POTUS's incompetence, the carnage he's helped inflict will be less.

In the first century after Europeans arrived in the Americas, up to 90 percent of indigenous people were exterminated. Germs did more killing than guns, and smallpox was a leading cause. In the first 80 years of the 20th century alone, at which time WHO announced its eradication, smallpox killed 300 million worldwide.

Since 1981, AIDS has killed 32 million. Thirty-eight million, including 1.2 million in America, are living with HIV now. The disease continues to kill 770,000 each year, the vast majority in resource-poor countries.

In 1899, the sixth cholera pandemic began in India, where in a year it killed 800,000. The seventh pandemic started in Indonesia in 1961 and continues to this day.

And who can forget the Black Death of 1347-1351, which killed maybe 50 million, half of Europe's population? Black Death, the moniker as old as Homer's monstrous Scylla, her mouths "full of black death," referred to the buboes, or swollen lymph nodes, that blackened the victim as the bacterium killed. Daniel Defoe's *A Journal of the Plague Year*, published in 1722, describes this bubonic plague in 1665 London, while Geraldine Brooks' novel *Year of Wonders* is set in an English village that same year.

Smallpox killed in a matter of weeks, the plague dispatched its victims in days, while cholera can claim the life of a healthy adult in six hours; all invoked more terror than COVID, perhaps part of the reason why some still refuse to take it seriously.

Across the globe, according to Worldometer, there have been more than 18 million cases of COVID, deaths from which will soon exceed 700,000.

Everything's relative.

What else might conservatives have a point about? Overland messengers heralded the advance of the plague; news of the Spanish Flu arrived by newspaper or radio; while cable channels carry COVID updates 24-7, stats shown in eye-catching displays, with added info a mere Google search away. Compared to past pandemics, we hear about our current plague constantly.

But hearing about the virus interminably hasn't been sufficient for all of us to "see" it. POTUS, for instance, sometimes acknowledges the "invisible enemy" even as he wants to, tries to, wish it away. There are people for whom the only way to envision the virus may be to witness, or hear about, its ravages on someone they know. In that Tulsa convention center, Herman Cain didn't see the virus he'd been dismissive of, the virus that caused his death.

HOW DOES THE
CORONAVIRUS SPREAD?

August 7

How does the coronavirus spread?

In Brazil, home to the world's second-highest COVID death toll next to the United States and home to a similarly arrogant and buffoonish president, the Amazon is a prime vehicle. In centuries past, European explorers sought gold, land, and converts, and brought with them the smallpox and measles that decimated indigenous groups. Today the river and its tributaries transport goods and industry to 30 million people scattered across eight countries, deep within forest that is otherwise impenetrable.

And as it did 500 years ago, the river brings disease. The six Brazilian cities with the highest COVID cases per capita sit on the banks of the Amazon. The virus has spread up and downstream from Manaus, the capitol of Amazonas state, traveling with families by dugout canoe and hitching a ride on boats carrying 100 or more passengers who sleep side-by-side at night. Boats carry medical personnel deep into the jungle, searching for people to test, other vessels deliver medicine, and boat ambulances take the sick from doctor-less villages to Manaus, a city of high rises and factories. In Manaus recently, daily deaths from the virus have surpassed 100, forcing the government to cut new burial grounds from dense forest, where workers lay coffins end-to-end in trenches in the freshly-turned earth.

How does the coronavirus spread?

In Brazil as well as in America, by an indifferent and incompetent president. Jair Bolsonaro, a right-wing populist in POTUS's mold, has compared COVID to a "measly flu." Brazilians, he's said, "never catch anything." They can "swim in raw sewage" and "nothing happens."

From his first days in power, Bolsonaro has made it clear that protecting indigenous communities isn't a priority. He's decreased their funding, whittled away at their protections, and encouraged illegal incursions into their lands. Indigenous Brazilians are six times more likely to contract the virus than whites are, echoing U.S. stats, where Native Americans are twice as likely to die from COVID as are whites.

How does the coronavirus spread?

In addition to transmission by respiratory droplets, it can be transmitted by aerosol. What's the difference?

Respiratory droplets consist of water vapor in which virus may be enmeshed. Infected patients cough or sneeze these droplets into the air—even talking or breathing can do the trick—where others may breathe them in. Because the droplets are denser than air, they tend to fall to the ground within a six-foot radius. Infection by inhalation of respiratory droplets is thought to be the main mode of transmission for both COVID and the flu.

Airborne particles—those capable of being transmitted through an airborne mechanism, like the measles virus, which is several times more contagious than COVID—are smaller than droplets, sometimes less than a micrometer. They're smaller because of less water vapor, which makes them less dense, so they can float in the air for hours before finally fluttering like snowflakes to the ground. Several groups of researchers have found COVID RNA hovering in the air several meters from infected patients. (*Genetic* material, not viable virus; if scientists succeed in isolating the latter, any remaining controversy about COVID being an airborne pathogen will disappear.)

Early in the pandemic, there was concern for COVID transmission via contaminated surfaces. Fox fomented this fear (if it scares your grandma and pisses off your grandpa, it's a Fox News story) and Dr. Oz whipped up hysteria. Not to pick on the TV personality excessively; I suspect all of us look back on behaviors in this pandemic that in retrospect seem too much. I no longer worry about clutching handrails on the stairs. At my age, I figure, a tumble is likelier than contracting COVID from a contaminated banister. That the virus can be viable for 72 hours on certain surfaces, imprinted months ago on susceptible minds, minds eager to learn how to stay safe, was established under *experimental* conditions. In real life, quantities of shed virus on inanimate objects are minuscule, droplets quickly desiccate, and COVID croaks. Researchers have yet to grow the virus from environmental samples in cell cultures designed for the task, nor has this mode of transmission been definitively documented.

But absence of evidence isn't evidence of absence. Stay humble, right? It's a *novel* virus. There's still a lot to learn!

So, given the above, what steps should you take to keep yourself safe, and which are superfluous?

COVID is a *respiratory* pathogen, infecting the nasal passages before invading the lungs. It's transmitted through the *air*. Coughing = sneezing > singing > talking > breathing, efficiency-wise. The longer your exposure, the higher your risk. I wouldn't have a conversation of more than a few sentences indoors within two meters if neither I nor my interlocutor wore a mask. Even before Gov. Evers' recent mandate, I put one on in any commercial enterprise. Other than twice with my family, when rain chased us indoors, I haven't dined inside a restaurant, though I've eaten on the decks of several, trying to stay six feet away from my friends.

I'm biking in groups again. But as much as I love the Green Bay Packers, I won't go to Lambeau to see them, not this season, if a season takes place. Though outside is much safer than in, all else being equal, until I'm vaccinated, even if wearing a mask, I'll avoid crowds.

Don't disinfect your mail before bringing it in or take off your work shoes before you walk in your house. It's not necessary, in my opinion, to wear gloves at the grocer's. There are more important things to worry about. The election, for instance.

Life has risks. It shouldn't be 100 percent safe. The unexamined life isn't worth living, but nor is the unlived life worth examining. Strive for prudence—e.g., on a national scale, an indoor mask mandate—but don't live in fear.

How does the coronavirus spread?

By dishonesty, including a press conference by lab-coat-clad physicians on the steps of the Supreme Court. After this video of "America's Frontline Doctors" was posted by Breitbart, POTUS tweeted references to it several times, followed by Don Junior, whose hereditary incapacity for critical thought made him call it a "must watch." The video quickly went viral, spreading more rapidly than COVID at a poultry-processing plant, amassing 14 million views on Facebook before the monopoly pulled it for "sharing false information about cures and treatments for Covid-19."

The company later said the hours that passed between the posting of the video and its removal "took longer than it should have." Among the lies told by a Dr. Stella Immanuel included "you don't need masks, there is a cure, it's called hydroxychloroquine, zinc, and azithromycin."

On her Facebook page, Dr. Immanuel describes herself as "God's battle axe and weapon of war." She claims that gynecologic problems can be caused by sex with demons. "Many women suffer from astral sex regularly," she says. "Astral sex"—in case you didn't know—"is the ability to project one's spirit man into the victim's body and have intercourse with it." After her video was yanked, she tweeted, "Hello Facebook put back my profile page and videos up or your computers will start crashing till you do. You are not bigger than God. I promise you. If my page is not back up face book will be down in Jesus name."

Every country has kooky docs. But only ours has a president kooky enough to not only endorse one, but also to amplify the misinformation in a McCarthy-esque way, leading more and more people (astrally) astray, contributing to more and more COVID casualties.

Words matter.

The *truth* matters.

How does the coronavirus spread?

By substandard public health, compared to other advanced countries. Historically, public health in the U.S. has received short shrift. It's chronically underfunded. POTUS doesn't perceive public health's significance and cares not a whit that he's kneecapped its vital mission.

Contact tracing is basic public health, at which the U.S. is failing miserably. There are only 42,000 contact tracers nationwide, less than 40 percent of what the CDC deems sufficient. In many areas where the virus is raging, local health departments can't begin to keep up.

In June, when casinos reopened in Las Vegas, local health officials foresaw the surge that has swamped local health departments.

"It's just impossible with the numbers that we are seeing," said Devin Raman, a senior disease investigator in the Southern Nevada Health District, which includes the city. Raman estimates her department has been able to contact only 25 to 40 percent of people with a positive test. "Right now, unfortunately, we're just trying to keep our heads above water."

On Alabama's hard-hit Gulf Coast, health departments are stretched so thin workers are telling test-positive patients to call contacts themselves.

"Everything is overwhelmed," said Rendi Murphree, Mobile County's disease surveillance director. "It is not going well."

Some epidemiologists describe U.S. contact tracing as too little, too late. "You don't clean up an oil spill with paper towels," says Harvard's Marc Lipsitch. POTUS's DHHS seems to agree. "It is really impossible to contact trace," said Brett Giroir, the Assistant Secretary for Health, until case numbers come down.

But WHO Chief Adhanom Ghebreyesus notes that the WHO stopped an Ebola outbreak in eastern Congo—despite an ongoing war—by tracing 25,000 contacts a day. "If any country is saying contract tracing is difficult, it is a lame excuse," he says. Small wonder, then, that POTUS, with his thin orange skin, has announced the United States will abandon the WHO.

Contrast the U.S. with Germany, blessed with a functional public health system and a competent chancellor. From the early days of the pandemic, contact tracing was collaborative, as repurposed municipal workers and medical students lent a hand. Today new daily cases in Germany, a country one-fourth our size, have dwindled to the hundreds and daily deaths to the single digits.

How does the coronavirus spread?

If not wearing a mask is a civil liberty, think of what proud and bare-faced POTUS fans, card-carrying members of his loyal base, think of contact tracing? Whatever happened to the responsibilities, rather than merely the rights, of being a citizen? Sure, I can swing my fist, the Ninth Amendment gives me the right, but my prerogative ends where your face begins.

"We get a variety of responses from yelling and hanging up, to telling us that they have already contacted all of their friends and will not give us their names," said Jen Freiheit, public health director in Wisconsin's Kenosha County.

Only in America.

Yesterday it was announced that an Apple and Google-designed app to inform you of possible COVID exposure would be trialed in Virginia. Such apps have been in place across the globe for several months; South Korea rolled out a mandatory app for its 52 million citizens in early March; today, the country reported 20 new cases and one new death.

How does the coronavirus spread?

What sustains the pandemic?

Pandemic, from the Greek. Pan = all, demos = people. Everyone is affected, and everyone needs to help.

Addendum: On Sept. 16, Florida researchers announced they'd isolated viable virus from the air of COVID patients' hospital rooms. The authors said, "Patients with respiratory manifestations of COVID-19 produce aerosols in the absence of aerosol-generating procedures (AGPs)"—bronchoscopy, airway intubation, and nebulizer treatments are examples of AGPs—"that contain viable SARS-CoV-2, and these aerosols may serve as a source of transmission of the virus."

PERVASIVE BIAS

August 12

Earlier this week I saw a patient who's also a friend, a retired professor in his seventies. Before I became his doctor, we'd fished and canoed together.

"Charlie" has shocks of gray hair that curl at the sides of a bald pate. Despite back surgeries and joint replacements, he continues to be remarkably active, ambling along trout streams in the spring and bird hunting in the fall.

A couple months ago Charlie told me he began to have chest pains. The pain was sharp and confined to the left side of his chest. It wasn't associated with physical activity. Usually, in fact, it came on at rest. The pain didn't travel to his arms, jaw, or back, and wasn't associated with nausea, sweating, or breathlessness. Nothing provoked the discomfort, and nothing reliably made it go away.

In POTUS's America, the patriarchy is alive and well, but men still die, on average, seven years before women do. (Death rates for heart disease between the sexes are both one in three; the average age of first heart attack for men is 65 while for women it's 72.)

Many conditions cause chest pain, including pulmonary embolism, a dissecting aortic aneurysm, arthritis where ribs meet sternum, and inflammation in the lining of the heart or lungs. To simplify this "differential diagnosis," doctors try to discern if the pain comes from the heart.

Patients are sorted into three categories: cardiac pain, caused by angina or heart attack; non-cardiac pain, precipitated by something else; and "atypical" chest pain, with features from both groups, in which case docs need more info to make up their minds.

Charlie's pain was non-cardiac, I thought. The discomfort was sharp—not the typical pressure linked to angina—and occurred at rest. The pain wasn't associated with other features worrisome for heart disease. And I couldn't conceive of him dropping dead, no longer able to fish, hunt, or care for his wife, who is chronically ill. I couldn't believe, didn't want to believe, that he might die.

But Charlie has diabetes, and his HDL, the "good" or protective cholesterol, runs low—risk factors for heart disease. What made me think he wouldn't have a heart attack? Because he's my friend, I had trouble wrapping my head around a worst-case scenario. I don't want my patients to die, of course, not a one, but the feeling may be stronger for patients who are also friends.

My problem was optimism bias, a cognitive prejudice toward a rosier outcome than is probable. Charlie, I reconsidered, had *atypical* chest pain. I ordered a treadmill stress test with radionuclide imaging. If it's normal, his risk of heart attack in the next few years will be minimal. If not, he'll see a cardiologist.

In 2004, at age 58, Bill Clinton had bypass surgery. His bad cholesterol three years earlier had been very high at 177—less than 100 is optimal—but Clinton wasn't taking a cholesterol medicine to lower his cardiac risk, the efficacy of which had been confirmed by many studies. Did optimism bias blind his doctors to the possibility that the patient who four years earlier had been the most powerful man on earth could develop heart disease?

Richard Nixon died from a stroke caused by atrial fibrillation, an irregular heart rhythm predisposing him to cardiac clots. The blood thinner warfarin could have prevented the clot that killed the former president, but he wasn't taking it. Did his doctors fall prey to the same cognitive error?

In medicine, doctors use cognitive shortcuts termed heuristics to home in on diagnoses, sometimes mere sentences into a patient's history. Usually, these heuristics don't lead them astray.

But sometimes they do. To ensure an accurate diagnosis, fast-thinking heuristics must yield to the hard work of thinking slowly, without which cognitive mistakes more readily take place. In representativeness bias, a physician is overly influenced by what is typically true. Availability bias occurs when a doctor, evaluating a new patient, puts too much weight on what he's recently seen. The elderly woman with fever and pain in the left lower quadrant of her abdomen? Maybe it's not another case of diverticulitis. Perhaps it's a kidney infection. In confirmation bias, after making a provisional diagnosis, a doctor gloms onto lab and x-ray data that corroborate his first impression while ignoring refuting evidence. Anchoring bias, which is similar, makes a doc reluctant to abandon his initial hunch.

Such biases aren't limited to medicine. In the dating world, how often do women keep seeing some ne'er-do-well guy? Why continue to anchor yourself to an anchor?

Concerning the pandemic, what cognitive biases may have worsened America's health? People are troubled by the thought of a patient with COVID presenting to the hospital short of breath and unable to be saved because of a shortage of ventilators (early on, the government appropriated $3 billion to build more ventilators), but they're not similarly distraught that social distancing, testing, and contact tracing weren't done sooner or more comprehensively, though the measures would have saved far more lives.

This bias has been called "the identifiable victim effect." We respond more aggressively to threats against individuals who we can more readily imagine to be friends and family than to hidden and future "statistical" deaths. Doctors also deal with this bias, not wanting anyone to die for want of a ventilator. (Some may think that prioritizing immediately threatened lives is rational, since there's less uncertainty than with policies designed to save invisible lives not now at risk.)

The identifiable victim effect overlaps with optimism bias, a hard-wired tendency, as discussed, to predict better outcomes than are typically seen. Early pandemic predictions modeled best-case, worst-case, and most-likely estimates, which reflected intrinsic uncertainty. Sound policy would have tried to minimize mortality by preventing worst-case scenarios, but instead we acted as if the best case would most likely occur.

POTUS in particular, whose most consistent COVID comment is that it will go away. (Many experts believe that, even with a vaccine produced and widely administered, the virus will become endemic, living with us in perpetuity.)

"Present" bias is an added concern. Even setting aside visible victims at imminent risk, humans prefer to save a life in the present more than a future life, one reason why Americans spend a mere 2.5 percent of their health care dollars on public health. (The bias also explains, at least in part, the difficulty instilling a sense of urgency to combat climate change.)

Finally, consider omission bias. A man who commits a crime is guiltier than a man who looks on and allows it to happen. (Think of the officer who murdered George Floyd and the others who watched him do it.) If policy makers don't provide enough ventilators and if clinicians design triage plans because of insufficient supplies, well, if these schemes are implemented, the responsible physicians and government officials may think themselves culpable for patients' deaths. Much easier psychologically for a person to evade blame for failure to enact policies to mitigate the virus's spread.

According to a recent essay in *JAMA*, a legacy of COVID could be that "future governments implement policies that reduce morbidity and mortality under worst-case rather than best-case scenarios, consider future harms as readily as present ones, and attend as strongly to hidden deaths as to visible lives." If this happens, the authors suggest optimistically, the pandemic might eventually serve "as a stimulus, paradoxically, to improve population health."

This seems unlikely in America, at least the America we live in now. But isn't it pretty to think so?

WILL IT EVER END?

August 19

"Will it ever end?" my patient asked. Though she meant the pandemic, her words could have referred to the tenure of the Conman-in-Chief, as our subsequent discussion made clear.

George Will is sanguine about POTUS's demise. Joe Biden's election, he says, will end "national nightmare 2.0," America's second domestic debacle in as many generations, Gerald Ford having proclaimed finis to the first. "Hell is truth recognized too late," writes Will, channeling Hobbes, and Americans will glimpse the fiery pits in the nick of time.

Hmm. Presidential polls are eerily comparable to four years ago, when a similarly overconfident E.J. Dionne stated that "women would save us" from the pussy-grabbing candidate, even before this particular peccadillo of his had been brought to light. (Though a majority of college-educated white women cast their votes for Clinton, white women overall favored her opponent.) POTUS spoke in Oshkosh earlier this week, while Biden won't even fly to Milwaukee to accept the Democratic nomination tomorrow night.

Last weekend, I bicycled through rural Wisconsin—from Eau Claire to Chippewa to Barron and Rusk Counties, before limping into Washburn County—where POTUS yard signs outnumbered Biden's 20:1. On Lake Chetek, where our group rehydrated at Gilligan's Tiki Bar, pontoons flew

POTUS flags over boisterous revelers, a scene repeated on Upper Long Lake as we picnicked at a friend's cottage at the end of our route.

Barack Obama won rural Wisconsin in 2008, but eight years later, these same voters deserted Hillary Clinton, who didn't campaign in the state. In 2016, Clinton received 238,000 fewer votes than Obama had four years earlier, while POTUS—the current one—roughly equaled Romney's tally.

In neighboring Minnesota, the Democratic Party is the DFL. Come on, Joe, win back those rural folks!

"When you and I are vaccinated," I told my patient.

Operation Warp Speed, the federal government's vaccine initiative, if not quite matching the Starship Enterprise's velocity, is outpacing the timelines of most virologists. Eight months into the pandemic, there are over 200 COVID vaccine candidates, with seven already in Phase 3 trials.

Vaccines teach the immune system to identify and block microorganisms. When targeting viruses, vaccines activate T-helper cells, which instruct B-cells to make antibodies that block viral replication. In addition, B cells tell T-killer cells to search out and destroy any virus-infected cell.

COVID is a single strip of RNA surrounded by a protein shell from which emerge the crown-shaped spikes that give the coronavirus—corona is crown in Latin—its family name; seven coronaviruses are known to infect humans. The spike proteins provide a convenient target for vaccine makers.

Thus far, Operation Warp Speed has awarded $9.5 billion to vaccine companies. Moderna has received $955 million for manufacturing scale up while also scoring a contract for an additional $1.525 billion upon delivery of 100 million vaccine doses. Pfizer's joint venture with BioNTech has secured $1.95 billion for the same number of doses; the companies haven't taken federal cash for scale up or R&D.

Moderna and Pfizer have mRNA vaccines in Phase 3 trials. To make an mRNA vaccine, RNA is emulsed within fat bubbles that penetrate cells, where it's transformed into the mRNA that directs production of spike protein, turning the cells into vaccine factories. Though the technology facilitates vaccine fabrication en masse, commercial use of it against any microorganism has yet to occur.

Viral-vectored vaccines use a virus engineered to be harmless to ferry vaccine into a cell. They, too, can churn vaccine out rapidly. One possible problem is people developing immunity to the viral vector, a big deal if booster doses become necessary.

The University of Oxford, in partnership with AstraZeneca, and CanSino Biologics, together with the Beijing Institute of Biotechnology, have viral-vectored vaccines in Phase 3 trials. AstraZeneca has agreed to deliver 300 million vaccine doses, at a cost of $1.2 billion, to the United States; $4/dose is the lowest cost in Operation Warp Speed's portfolio. 800 million doses are currently under contract for 330 million people in the United States, the redundancy owing to the probability that some vaccine makers won't successfully deliver product in acceptable time.

No surprise that CanSino hasn't been offered a U.S. contract. Chinese companies can't be trusted! Not to fight the *Chinese* virus! No POTUS-supporting, science-bashing conservative would accept the risk! As we'll see, even with a vaccine made in America, Republicans are skeptical.

A third approach involves a weakened or inactivated virus capable of stimulating an immune response but not of causing infection; the Salk polio vaccine is a prototype. Two issues: manufacturing is time-consuming, which makes speedy vaccine production all but impossible; and the three companies in Phase 3 trials are all Chinese.

If you're desperate to be vaccinated, you could move to Russia. Despite being tested in less than 100 people, the country recently approved its viral-vectored vaccine for widespread use. Russian medical workers can line up to receive it by the end of the month, and the country intends to start mass inoculations in October. (China won the race to make its citizens guinea pigs, approving the CanSino vaccine for its military back in June.)

Moderna's Phase 3 trial is enrolling 30,000 people across America, 20,000 receiving the vaccine and 10,000 placebo. Oxford's trial will also recruit 30,000 volunteers. Why are these large-scale trials important? Even in studies of this magnitude, researchers will discover side effects only if they happen at a rate of more than 1 in 5,000.

A side effect in 1 in 10,000 would fly under the radar, so if the vaccine killed one in 10,000 recipients, for example, scientists won't know. In this theoretical scenario, if 300 million Americans got such a vaccine, 30,000 would die from it. (The tradeoff might be acceptable vis a vis preventable deaths, but most people, weighing immediate harm vs. future benefit, wouldn't take the risk. In the event, the FDA would pull the vaccine.)

After a successful Phase 3 trial, the FDA typically signs off on a vaccine. How often, after FDA approval, is a vaccine removed from the market? A recent study in the *Annals of Internal Medicine* looked at every vaccine approved by the FDA between 1996 and 2015. Just one in 57 was yanked, a rotavirus vaccine, because of an unusual intestinal complication, not an increased risk of death.

Earlier in the pandemic, epidemiologists estimated we'd have herd immunity when 70 to 80 percent of the population had either been exposed to the virus or vaccinated. Current estimates are lower, slightly under 50 percent. Good news, because many Americans are loathe to line up for a vaccine.

According to a recent Gallup poll, if an FDA-approved vaccine was available free of charge, 35 percent of Americans would refuse to take it. The difference along party lines was striking: 81 percent of Democrats would be vaccinated, while 53 percent of Republicans would decline.

How long will immunity from a vaccine last? No one knows, because they're still being trialed. The CDC suggests that exposure to COVID confers three months of immunity, but according to a recent study in the *New England Journal of Medicine*, half of the antibody mounted against mild infections is gone in little more than a month.

Scientists aren't even thinking about eradicating the coronavirus; smallpox remains the only virus in world history to have been consigned to that justified fate. Most likely, COVID will become endemic, circulating in (hopefully) low levels. Now and then, the virus will rear its ugly head in clusters, where the world's most destitute and thus least likely to be vaccinated will continue to be at risk. There's a good chance that every autumn, you'll get a COVID booster with your flu vaccine.

If only we could vaccinate against unreason, against blind faith, against unwillingness to care for our neighbor, against an inability to see that he or she may neither look like us nor live nearby.

PUT ON YOUR FUCKING MASK!

September 5

"Put on your fucking mask!"

The words were spat at me, if one can spit from beneath a mask, by a runner on the Golden Gate Bridge. He was fit, clipping along, 50s-ish, bound for San Francisco, while my wife and I walked toward Marin, out and then back on the famous expanse.

Smoke from wildfires had greeted us the night before upon our arrival, but the smell wasn't evident now. The wind whipped across the bridge, gusting to 30 mph, blowing my wife's long blond hair in front of her face. The bridge's rust-colored towers were hidden in fog, parts peaking out, for an instant, before fading away. Sailboats plied the bay below, safely distanced from commercial ships. Foghorns bellowed.

You're never alone on the Golden Gate Bridge, though throughout its history, hundreds must have felt as if they were before climbing past the railing and plunging to their deaths. Signs encourage anyone considering suicide to text 741741; a safety net to catch would-be jumpers keeps getting delayed; some oppose the aesthetics, while others argue that, concerning suicide, where there's a will there's a way.

The runner stared me down before telling me off. I'm not sure why he singled me out, passing everyone else with an uncovered face in respectful silence. I was wearing a Wisconsin Public Radio t-shirt. Was I a Badger State voter who'd helped ensconce POTUS on Pennsylvania Avenue? My hair is a longish and disheveled gray, while my wife is very pretty. Did he wonder how a man like me ended up with a woman like her? Was he jealous the gods had prescribed such a fate? Doubtful, but still.

Why was he pissed? Running, in my experience, tends to mellow a guy out. Perhaps, in a This-is-Water way, he'd had a bad day. Maybe his wife had left him. Perhaps a child was getting chemotherapy. Maybe earlier that morning he'd been in line at a 7-Eleven, waiting to pay for the Red Bull he'd slam before pounding the pavement, and a shaggy-haired man who resembled me was taking *forever* to buy an assortment of lottery tickets—mega millions, scratchers, daily 4s—and my antagonist had worked himself into a stew. Though not likely, to paraphrase David Foster Wallace, nor was it impossible.

A long line of pedestrians stretched out ahead of us, some several abreast, while helmeted cyclists pedaled past, perhaps half of each group wearing masks; only later did I learn that Gov. Gavin Newsome had mandated masks for anyone outside of their home. Ordinance-breaking aside, with the high winds on top of the bridge, the chance of a symptomless me passing the virus to the outraged runner, in the two or three seconds it took him to jog by, was less than him falling flat on his face and sustaining a brain bleed while he turned his head to admonish me. Politically, more likely than not, we were allies, but the mask kerfuffle kept either of us from noticing.

This incident, on the first of 10 days in California, was our only run in with mask-related animosity. To the contrary, people we encountered— trekking on Yosemite's trails, strolling through the coastal redwoods of Muir Woods, and tasting wine in Napa and Sonoma vineyards—were unfailingly polite. In the forest, when someone approached, if masks had slipped below chins, they were lifted to cover noses and mouths. You sensed that, regarding COVID in California, compared to in Wisconsin, there was a one-for-all and all-for-one mentality. As Newsome has said, government can't solve the problem all by itself.

At least in the Bay Area, citizens have responded, to good effect. San Francisco County, population 900,000, has had only 9,600 COVID cases contributing to 83 deaths. Its caseload per capita is roughly half of the USA's as a whole, while its death rate of 92/million is less than 1/5 of the nation's 572/million, a ratio increasing by 3 deaths/million Americans each day.

Why did we travel to California? What gave us the right? Didn't I know that California had had more COVID cases than any other state? If I wasn't concerned about my own health and welfare, what about my wife's? If I contracted COVID and unwittingly brought it home? To my patients or 90-year-old parents?

I had no business in California. No meetings to attend, no over-priced real estate to try and procure. Family obligations? Not really, though my wife's son and girlfriend joined us for the wine-tasting part of the trip, and my sister and her husband, who live in Marin County, graciously hosted us our final two nights. (Though *they're* careful, and *we're* careful, the four of us together, regarding masks and social distancing, could have been more fastidious; it's a numbers game, the odds of this or that; we're a small family, just me and my sister, who I see infrequently; we rationalize our behaviors, or justify them, as the case may be.)

The COVID pandemic is *interesting*, not least on an ethical front. What are my responsibilities to my fellow citizens? How do I ensure that they're safe?

We know more now than we did six months ago. Early on, shelter at home was a blunt but effective tool to keep the virus at bay. Fortunately, it's no longer necessary. If everyone wore a mask within an enclosed public space, and if large gatherings anywhere were verboten, if bars in hot spots were forced to close, or did so out of a sense of responsibility, transmission of COVID would sharply decrease. We'd still have to worry about family members—and friends, and workers on lunch breaks—infecting each other, but it would be a great start.

How does this relate to travel? Is it ethical? Is it safe?

A good friend who's more risk-averse than me won't fly until he's vaccinated. Does science support his decision? Early in the pandemic, the few times passengers symptomatic with COVID were known to have flown, no cases of in-air transmission were discovered. Now, on some airliners, middle seats aren't sold. We flew on Delta, while Alaskan, Hawaiian, Southwest, and Jet Blue have followed suit. In addition, hepa filters on Boeing aircraft trap more than 99.9 percent of microorganisms. Mandatory masking adds an additional, and in my view sufficient, safety level. Universal masking, combined with social distancing, transforms airports and car rental agencies into the equivalent of your local Menard's—you're merely more familiar with the latter if, like most Americans, you haven't flown since the pandemic began. In most California venues, indoor dining is prohibited. We ate outside, as in Wisconsin—while we can, while the weather permits. A Mobil station here or there is the same. All in all, I felt safer in California, which presents a more unified front against Covid-19.

When we're scared, we hunker down, build walls both real and metaphorical, trying to enhance our sense of security. The unknown—and the other, as we've seen through a summer of racial justice protests, where POTUS harangues on this other-wariness, maliciously trying to spin it to his political advantage—makes us afraid. Fear of the unknown explains much of why people are foregoing travel, while fear of the other permits policy makers to implement travel bans, one nation upon another, which have been widespread since the pandemic began.

Back in January, when the first COVID cases popped up in the United States, the WHO inveighed against travel bans, arguing that they disrupt trade, including the supply chains whose importance the pandemic soon magnified. More to the point, the WHO stated, they don't work.

In a 2014 paper, the WHO studied 23 outbreaks of pandemic influenza and concluded the following, using mathematical modeling:

Air travel restrictions in *all* affected countries may delay the spread of a pandemic by two to three weeks.

These restrictions have minimal impact on the magnitude of pandemics, typically reducing attack rates by *less than 0.02 percent.*

The more transmissible the influenza viral strain, the less effective are international—or internal, within a country—travel bans; since COVID is more transmissible than the flu, travel restrictions for COVID would be expected to be less useful than they are for the flu, a hypothesis consistent with subsequent history; the small island nations of New Zealand and Iceland are possible exceptions, though they also relied heavily on basic public health tactics—test, trace, and isolate, a trio the U.S. still refuses to take seriously— to bring COVID under control.

Such restrictions would not prevent the introduction of influenza into *any* given country. (all italics mine.)

The WHO paper looked at flu outbreaks before and up to the H1N1 pandemic of 2009. Since then, the world has only become more interconnected; it's useful to remember that the pandemic of 1918, before the advent of commercial air travel, had no problem engulfing the world.

It goes without saying that POTUS isn't burdened by profound scientific understanding, nor do the dictates of science affect his reasoning. Instead, COVID gave him cover to express his xenophobia through travel bans, though irony abounds. Europe needs protection—if travel bans could truly protect—from us more than the obverse, and the closure of the Canadian-American border, if it safeguards anyone, advantages our neighbors to the north.

Why did the masked runner on the Golden Gate Bridge yell at me? Did fear contribute to his outburst? Was it justified? Since I wasn't from California, did he judge me more harshly than he might have otherwise?

Probably not. But maybe he—and everyone else, including me, especially now, when many but by no means all of us are confronting America's ongoing racism, slavery's legacy—ought to be less inclined to think that an unknown other poses a threat.

Addendum: On Sept. 18, the CDC reported that two flight attendants were infected by one of two passengers, a husband and wife who developed COVID symptoms March 10, the day their flight, departing from Boston, arrived in Hong Kong. Genetic viral sequencing proved that the passengers had infected the flight attendants.

Two additional studies published the same week—one involved a March 1 Vietnam Airlines flight from London to Hanoi, while the other looked at travel on 18 international flights to and from Greece between Feb. 26 and March 9—suggested that in-flight transmission of the virus had likely occurred.

None of these studies noted whether or not flight attendants or passengers wore masks. However, it's doubtful that passengers in the studies, early on in the pandemic, wore masks, and most airlines didn't start mandating masks for flight attendants until April, at the earliest.

RACE MATTERS

September 9

"You saw the same tape as I saw," said POTUS, referring to Kyle Rittenhouse, the 17-year-old who'd transported two AR-15s to Kenosha, where he killed two BLM protestors. "And he was trying to get away from them. I guess it looks like he fell and then they very violently attacked him. I guess he was in very big trouble. He probably would have been killed."

Of Rittenhouse, Rep. Thomas Massie said, "He also exhibited tremendous restraint and presence and situational awareness. He didn't empty a magazine into a crowd. There were people around him who could have caused him harm, but as soon as they showed any sign of retreat or nonaggression, he did not shoot them." The Kentucky Republican has served in Congress since 2012, never garnering less than 62 percent of the vote. In the "prolife" party, preemptive killing is becoming a routine rationale for taking a human life.

In the late 19th century, Booker T. Washington put the Tuskegee Institute on the map. On his fund-raising travels, he set white audiences at ease by sharing southern "darky" jokes. In return for this one-man minstrel show, those whites wrote him checks. In Ibram Kendi's words, "Washington somehow demeaned Black people as stupid for an hour and then received donations to educate those same stupid people."

In 1901, Washington released his book *Up From Slavery* to great acclaim. Later that year, on Oct.16, President Theodore Roosevelt, newly sworn in after William McKinley's assassination, invited to dinner "the most distinguished member of his race in the world." Though blacks had built the presidential living quarters and had served there ever since, none had ever dined with a president.

The uproar was swift and furious. South Carolina Senator Ben Tillman: "The action of President Roosevelt in entertaining that nigger will necessitate our killing a thousand niggers in the South before they learn their place again."

Roosevelt learned his lesson and never again asked a black person to dine with him. But the South kept hurling abuse at him. Later that month, Roosevelt officially named his new dwelling place the White House, but the verbal onslaught continued.

Give Send Go, the "#1 Christian Crowdfunding Site," has raised, as of this writing, from more than 11,000 donors, $479,000 for Rittenhouse's legal defense, rallying the troops with the following: "Kyle Rittenhouse just defended himself from a brutal attack by multiple members of the far-left group ANTIFA." (No evidence ties ANTIFA to his August 25 killings.) "The experience was undoubtedly a brutal one, as he was forced to take two lives to defend his own."

Donations are pouring in. Recent comments from his benefactors, reported in sequence:

"Praying for you Kyle! You were certainly raised right!"

"Kyle, stand strong in the Lord Jesus."

"God bless America! God bless Kyle and his family!! We need more Patriots like him!!! We stand by you!!!!!"

"Kyle, we are praying for you, God bless you."

"G-d Bless Kyle, may he obtain justice for his self-defense against the mob. May G-d be kind to him in Heaven regardless."

"Pray for America and it's flip flopped morals."

"Keep your head up Kyle—the silent majority is with you!"

"Kyle, a lot of America knows the real story & are praying for you & your family. May God Bless & keep you!"

"God bless you & your family."

"Praying for u, stay strong by the Lord's grace."

In 1915 Woodrow Wilson became the first president to screen a movie at the White House, choosing *The Birth of a Nation*, a silent film based on Thomas Dixon's novel *The Clansmen*. The film ahistorically depicted Reconstruction as an era of corrupt black supremacists scaring the bejesus out of innocent whites. In the climax, a black male rapist—played by a white actor in blackface—pursues a white woman into the woods until she jumps to her death.

"Lynch him, lynch him!" shouted Houston moviegoers. That year, nearly 100 black men were lynched. At movie's end, the victim's brother organizes Klansmen to regain control of southern society, and a white Jesus blesses the triumph of white supremacy as the film concludes.

By January 1916, more than 3 million had watched the film in New York City alone. For two decades, it was the highest grossing movie in America.

According to a 2019 nationwide survey, 86 percent of white evangelical Protestants and 70 percent of both Catholics and mainline Protestants say the Confederate flag is more a symbol of Southern pride than of racism; nearly two-thirds of white Christians say the killings of black men by the police are isolated incidents instead of a broader pattern of mistreatment; and more than 60 percent of white Christians don't agree that "generations of slavery and discrimination have created conditions that make it difficult for blacks to work their way out of the lower class."

In his new book *White Too Long*, Robert P. Jones, the head of the Public Religion Research Institute, a non-partisan polling and research organization, states, startlingly, that "the more racist attitudes a person holds, the more likely he or she is to identify as a white Christian," a perspective that stands in sharp contrast to that of religiously unaffiliated whites.

"If you were recruiting for a white supremacist cause Sunday morning," Jones says, "you'd likely have more success hanging out in the parking lot of an average white Christian church than approaching whites sitting out services at the local coffee shop."

Faith, hope, and love, says First Corinthians. Please forgive me, but faith seems an unworthy companion of the latter two. Faith sometimes shares the stage with prejudice, commingles with certitude, and is "strengthened" by suspending critical thought. Does belief in a particular creed—or religious faith in general—cause more problems than it solves?

In 1939 MGM released *Gone with the Wind*, based on Margaret Mitchell's Pulitzer Prize-winning novel. The film smashed box office records and racked up 10 Academy Awards. The loyal and loving Mammy, both a fiction and a stereotype, became one of the most adored characters in Hollywood history. "By enjoying her servitude," wrote political scientist Melissa Harris-Perry in a 2011 review of the movie, "Mammy acts as a healing salve for a nation ruptured by the sins of racism."

Twelve Years a Slave ain't *Gone with the Wind*. The 2013 Oscar winner, which showed the horrific reality of slavery rather than a love affair with the antebellum South, made $187 million worldwide, including $56 million domestically. In its day, *Gone with the Wind* raked in $400 million, or $3.44 billion in 2014 dollars, still the highest (inflation-adjusted) grossing film of all time.

Kyle Rittenhouse has become a darling of right-wing media. Tucker Carlson wonders why anyone should be surprised that "17-year-olds with rifles decided they had to maintain order when no one else would." Conservative provocateur Ben Shapiro notes that Joseph Rosenbaum, the unarmed man chasing and lunging toward Rittenhouse, who the teenager then shot in the head, was a registered sex offender, while Anthony Huber, shot in the chest by Rittenhouse as Huber attempted to subdue him with his skateboard (after multiple demonstrators identified Rittenhouse as the shooter), had a felony conviction for domestic abuse.

According to blogger Robert Stacy McCain, "That's the ultimate 'play a stupid game, win a stupid prize.' You're running, chasing somebody down. The person you're chasing has a rifle. What did you expect?"

"Amazing marksmanship," McCain adds. "Given a sufficient supply of ammunition, Rittenhouse could have wiped out every Antifa thug in Kenosha."

"R.I.P., sex offender," the blogger concluded.

Does having a police record devalue a human life?

In 1982, President Ronald Reagan said, "We must mobilize all our forces to stop the flow of drugs into this country" and to "brand drugs such as marijuana exactly for what they are—dangerous."

Drug crime was declining, only 2 percent of people thought drugs to be America's most pressing problem, but no matter.

In 1985, there were 757,000 inmates in federal and state prisons. Thirty-five percent were black, and 64 percent white (including Hispanics). In 1986, with broad bipartisan support, Reagan signed the Anti-Drug Abuse Act. (In the Senate, the vote was 97-2, and in the House, 392-16.)

One provision prescribed a mandatory minimum of five years in prison for anyone caught with five grams of crack cocaine—used mostly by poor people who are disproportionately black—while the mostly white and rich dealers or users of powder cocaine had to be caught with 500 grams to warrant the same sentence.

In August 1994, President Bill Clinton signed The Violent Crime Control and Law Enforcement Act. The $30 billion bill created dozens of new federal capital crimes, imposed mandatory life sentences for certain three time offenders, and led to the largest increase in prisoners in U.S. history, most of whom were incarcerated following convictions for non-violent drug offenses.

By 2000, blacks comprised 62.7 percent of drug offenders in state prisons—blacks represent 13 percent of the population, then and now—compared to 36.7 percent for whites, though the National Survey on Drug Abuse in that year reported an equivalent 6.4 percent of both blacks and whites used illegal drugs. In 2000, the total prison population had swelled to over 1.3 million: 470,000 white, 620,000 black, and 217,000 Hispanic.

Since then, racial disparities in convictions and sentencing, though persistent, have diminished. Last year, Adam Geld, CEO of the Council on Criminal Justice, referring to 2000-2016 pre-POTUS data, said, "If the perception is that this is a bad problem getting worse, the reality is it's going from worse to bad." The decline coincides with extensive marketing of Oxycontin by Purdue Pharma in the late 1990s and early 2000s, jumpstarting an opioid epidemic that mostly affects whites.

Joe Biden visited Kenosha Sept. 3, two days after POTUS. He talked by phone with Jacob Blake, who remains hospitalized, and met with Blake's family for 90 minutes. Blake's mother led the group in prayer for her son's recovery. Afterwards, Blake's attorney said, "The vice president told the family that he believes the best of America is in all of us and that we need to value all our differences as we come together in America's great melting pot. It was very obvious that Vice President Biden cared, as he extended to Jacob a sense of humanity, treating him as a person worthy of consideration and prayer."

Does POTUS believe we have a problem with race? If so, does he think it inheres in centuries of white mistreatment of blacks? Does he get that Joseph Rosenbaum and Anthony Huber weren't killed out of self-defense or because a 17-year-old was trying to protect commercial property from being vandalized, but because a policeman shot an unarmed black man seven times in the back?

Most black people won't bet their lives on it.

LONG HAULERS

September 14

Last week I saw a patient with COVID, a young man I'd never met. He wasn't acutely ill, but four months after becoming infected, the virus yet damaged his health. Isaiah—not his real name—was in his late 20s, with long blond hair, a like-colored beard, and a gentle mien. From behind black-rimmed glasses, blue eyes took me in. He wore shorts and a t-shirt commemorating a field trip he'd taken years earlier as a student at UW-Eau Claire, a tour of civil rights sites including Selma and Birmingham.

Isaiah is a cashier—an essential worker—at a local convenience store. He was sickened in April, before the store mandated masks for staff or customers. He had no idea who'd infected him.

His first symptom was unexplained pain, as if a vise gripped the right side of his chest, sometimes migrating to his collarbone or descending to his lower ribs. The constant squeezing he could tolerate, but stabs that came out of the blue sometimes dropped him to his knees. Because he didn't have health insurance, he endured the pain.

A week later, Isaiah developed typical COVID symptoms of cough and fever and shortness of breath. He lost his sense of smell. Profound fatigue swallowed him up, confining him to his apartment. Fortunately for his finances, he wasn't sick enough to be hospitalized.

Though his cough and fever disappeared in days, exhaustion lingered. When he returned to work, a quick walk across the store could leave him gasping for breath. Compared to his childhood asthma, the air hunger felt different, without the musical wheezing he'd had as a youth.

Convenience store colleagues pointed out errors of which he'd not been aware. He chalked them up to inadequate rest, despite sleeping 10 or 12 hours a night. To Isaiah, it seemed as if his weariness had crept into his brain.

Most bothersome, his chest pain continued. Neither ibuprofen nor heat or ice put a dent in it.

A lung CT scan six weeks after his diagnosis revealed the ground glass opacities that are classic for COVID. There was no sign of a pulmonary embolism, a blood clot that might have moved to his lungs, to which COVID patients are predisposed. Young people with the virus sometimes develop myocarditis, inflammation of the heart muscle, but tests for this and other cardiac conditions came back negative. His symptoms stumped a cardiologist, who thought they arose from the bones, joints, or muscles of his chest wall.

When I met Isaiah, he still had constant chest pain punctuated by lightning-like jabs. His lassitude was less, but only marginally. Riding his bike around town at a casual pace still left him breathless. In recent weeks, a new symptom had begun: pounding headaches brought on by the least physical toil.

His exam was normal. Clear lungs, regular heart sounds. But when my nurse took a brisk walk with him around the unit, his oxygen saturation dropped to 90 (healthy levels for a young person remain in the high 90s) and he labored to breathe.

A review of *Up To Date*, our go-to online resource, failed to suggest the cause of his pain. I agreed with the cardiologist that it probably came from his chest wall, though I didn't know why. I prescribed a high dose of naproxen, an anti-inflammatory, figuring that whatever was causing his pain, inflammation lay at its root.

The inflammation accompanying the immune response to acute COVID infection may make patients go quickly downhill; the virus attacks the air sacs of the lungs, which the immune reaction to infection further inflames, so that oxygen delivery is impaired. Clinical trials have shown that the potent steroid dexamethasone, another anti-inflammatory, affords a survival advantage to COVID patients who are critically ill.

Maybe the virus had inflamed Isaiah's ribs, or the muscles between them. Perhaps this irritation persists.

We're dealing with a novel virus, an unheard of microbe less than a year ago. Doctors and scientists can infer by analogy with the six other coronaviruses known to infect humans—SARS could be lethal, MERS often is, while four lead to nothing worse than the common cold—but these hypotheses are merely educated guesses.

What else don't we know much about? The chronic complications of infection. After all, in the United States, the pandemic is only six months old. Besides stroke, which is common, other neurological complications include encephalitis or encephalopathy, the former caused by brain infection and the latter by a pro-inflammatory cytokine storm that destroys the brain. Less severe central nervous system involvement is common. COVID infection of olfactory nerves, besides nixing sense of smell, may be the conduit by which the virus invades the brain, subsequently infecting other neurons and impairing cognition, subtly or not. The blood-brain barrier is more readily disrupted in older patients, another means for the virus to enter the brain, perhaps a partial explanation for increased mortality in the elderly.

Myocarditis and myocardial infarction can lead to congestive heart failure. Acute kidney injury may turn into chronic disease. Livers sometimes take a hit; the worse the acute illness, the poorer they fare. Clots form in arteries and cause gangrene. Clots form in veins and float to the lungs.

A study from Italy, evaluating patients hospitalized with COVID a mean of two months after their symptoms began, found only one in eight had made a full recovery. More than half reported fatigue; over 40 percent cited breathlessness; upwards of a quarter had joint pain; and more than one in five had ongoing chest pain. Lung damage explains shortness of breath, but mechanisms for the other three remain elusive.

A CDC study found that 14 to 21 days after testing positive 35 percent of COVID outpatients—people not sick enough to need to be hospitalized—had ongoing symptoms, most commonly fatigue, cough, headache, and shortness of breath. Two to three weeks into their illnesses, 26 percent of 18 to 34-year-olds hadn't wholly recovered their health.

The combination of fatigue, brain fog, headache, and malaise following exercise has been termed "post-COVID syndrome."

In addition to my new patient, how many more Americans will eventually be diagnosed with it?

WHAT CAN WE LEARN FROM CANADA?

September 16

On Sept. 11, for the first time in six months, Canada reported no new deaths from COVID. The same day, the country reported 702 new cases. (Canada's population of 38 million is 1/9 of ours.) Yesterday, the United States reported 52,081 new COVID cases, the most in more than a month, and 1422 new deaths. Why the big difference?

According to Dr. Larry Lutwick, senior infectious disease specialist at Mayo-Eau Claire, "In Canada, they listen to their public health specialists." Lutwick continued, "I have a friend in Toronto. When they had SARS, in 2003, they did what they needed to and quickly shut it down." Referring to pandemic management in the United States, he said, "It's embarrassing."

On Aug. 7, in Millinocket, Maine, in violation of a state mandate limiting indoor gatherings to 50 or less, 65 people attended a wedding. One celebrant worked at Maplecrest Rehabilitation and Living Center in the town of Madison.

Now 176 COVID cases have been linked to the wedding, including seven deaths. Six of the dead were residents of Maplecrest. None of the decedents attended the wedding, which has also been linked to an outbreak at the York County jail. Both the jail and the nursing home are more than 100 miles, in different directions, from Millinocket.

On Sept. 13, POTUS held an indoor rally in Henderson, Nev. An esti-mated 5,600 diehards—though death may come more easily to them and their loved ones than they could have conceived—crammed into the venue, and up to 20,000 more amassed outside.

Behind POTUS at the podium sat masked supporters on the dais, to be captured by journalists' cameras, while there were few masks amongst the throng he addressed. (From the now notorious Skagit, Wash., choir rehearsal six months ago, where one singer unwittingly infected 52 of 60 colleagues, including two who died, we got our first inkling that singing—or shouting or chanting—more readily transmits COVID than talking or breathing.) In one ironic Henderson pic, a single supporter is wearing a mask, black with white letters spelling TRUMP. Surrounding him, some in the audience, most also white and male, scream their lungs out for the Conman-in-Chief.

"And we also believe," POTUS declaimed, "that if you murder a police officer, you should receive the death penalty and that's something that's very important."

The crowd chanted, "U.S.A.!"

"They don't like my personality, but I hate to say it, I'm what you need. I'm what you need. It's true." Audience, shouting, "We love you! We love you!"

"You burn the flag, you go to jail for one year. I would love to see it. I would love to see it. I would love to see it."

"U.S.A., U.S.A., U.S.A!"

Referring to COVID, POTUS said, "Other countries are doing terribly. Did you see the statistics of us compared to other countries? Us compared to Europe? Us compared..."

We have, and he has not.

"We have done an incredible job," he said.

There's an ironic truth to this claim, as incredible means impossible to believe. Incredible, really, for the most powerful person in the world to have so thoroughly mismanaged the pandemic. Incredible that the occupant of the highest office in the land is a psychopathic narcissist willing to sacrifice lives at the altar of his ego.

In Kenosha two weeks ago, at a roundtable meeting with law enforcement, local officials, and business owners, POTUS told participants they could remove their masks "if you feel more comfortable doing so." "Look at how fast you took that off," he said to one. At the end of the meeting, no face was covered.

Last night, at a town hall from Philadelphia's National Constitution Center, POTUS acknowledged that the pandemic has been his presidency's biggest challenge. Moderator George Stephanopoulos asked him, "Could you have done more to stop it?"

"I don't think so," POTUS said.

He denied that he'd downplayed the virus and then said, "We're going to be okay and it is going away," even, he added, "without the vaccine."

Not only was it impossible for him to have done more to limit the carnage, our vainglorious leader thinks he's saved millions of lives. "I think what I did by closing up the country (limiting flights from China on Jan. 31), I think I saved two, maybe two and half (million), maybe more than that, lives."

When a questioner asked POTUS why he only infrequently wore a mask, "I do wear them when I have to and when I'm in hospitals and other locations" was all he said.

Also two weeks ago, Dr. Theresa Tam, Canada's Chief Public Health Officer, said that if someone chooses to have sex outside of their bubble, they should avoid kissing and wear a mask; compliance isn't projected to be high. Since July 13, Canada has recorded only 400 deaths, an interval in which more than 60,000 Americans have died. Once again, why such a disparity?

According to an essay in *JAMA* last month:

1. Canada has less political polarization than the U.S., and the pandemic, for the most part, hasn't been politicized.

2. Despite differences in political affiliation, the federal and provincial governments have cooperated.

3. There's less mistrust of science and public health.

4. Though some leaders initially misjudged the virus, none have doubted, since the end of March, the seriousness of its challenges. The authors, two Toronto physicians, thought this observation their most significant.

Most of us, when we look in the mirror, at least some of the time, don't like what we see. Unfortunately for America, when POTUS stares at his image, true love returns his gaze, blinding him to reality.

LOVE IS ALL WE NEED.
OR IS IT?

September 24

Two of the best writers in the United States are black female immigrants. The Nigerian Chimamanda Adichie, a MacArthur fellow and author of *We Should All be Feminists*, won the National Book Critics Circle Award in 2013 for her novel *Americanah*. Edwidge Danticat, who hails from Haiti, won the same award in 2007 for her autobiographical *Brother, I'm Dying*.

Adichie last saw her 88-year-old father in early March. On June 9, she spoke with him by video. He felt a bit unwell, was sleeping poorly, but told her not to worry. She kept the chat brief so he could rest. He died the next day. When her brother called to tell her, relates Adichie in a recent *New Yorker* article, she came undone.

How can this be, she wonders? Just that afternoon, her father had read the newspaper, talked to his son about shaving before the following day's appointment with a kidney specialist, and spoken by phone with another daughter, a doctor, about his lab results. "But there he is," Adichie says. Her brother Okey is "holding a phone over my father's face, and my father looks asleep, his face relaxed, beautiful in repose. Our Zoom call is beyond surreal, all of us weeping and weeping and weeping, in different parts of the world, looking in disbelief at the father we adore lying still on a hospital bed."

The family hasn't been able to plan a funeral. Nigeria's airports remain closed to international travel.

Danticat lives among Miami's Haitian diaspora. In a recent essay in the *New York Review of Books*, she says, "My neighbor died recently. I saw the ambulance arrive. The red and blue strobes bounced off every glass surface on both sides of our block. She was 80 years old and ambulances had come for her before."

Danticat continues, "When my mother died of ovarian cancer in our house, this neighbor came over to sit with us that same night. She came over to pray with us when my mother was near death. We attended the same small church and sometimes I gave her and her slightly younger sister a ride home. She loved to hand out cookies and hard candy to the kids at church. She cooed over both my daughters when they were just days old."

The Haitian-American mourns the passing of her mourning rituals, "the home visits, the festive wakes, the funerals, and post-burial repasts." She and her husband and their two daughters live with her mother-in-law, who told her that in dreams, a feast means death. Is death, Danticat muses, a form of celebration in another realm?

Recently at dusk, she sat with her family beside the ocean, the first time in weeks they'd been allowed at the beach. The luminous sky, as if the clouds had been set aflame, reminded her "that colors, like viruses, could mutate. That afternoon, it was as if the sky had become a colossal color-field painting, with layers upon layers of hues and shades, pigments and shapes, dipping into the horizon."

Why did this occur? A storm in the Sahara Desert had sent a plume of dust all the way to Miami. Out of chaos and destruction, phoenix-like, beauty appeared.

The Catholic priest I've worked with in Port-au-Prince, Father Rick Frechette, observes that the facial muscles used in crying and laughing are the same. Sorrow's depth may mirror the height of previous joy, as if yin and yang balance out. If we've never experienced joy, maybe it's not possible to truly grieve; perhaps when we're sad, we ought to give thanks.

But I'm not sure. I saw a patient last week, a retired history professor, who said that although the protests following the death of George Floyd may have been justified, Black Lives Matter has become "an ideology." "I am not racist. None of the professors I taught with are racist. America is the least racist country on earth," he declared, echoing POTUS, who said to a questioner during his town hall a week ago, "Well, I hope there's not a race problem," before abruptly changing the subject.

Our state representative lives just down the street. Although our politics couldn't be more dissimilar—he introduced himself two years ago when he first ran for office as a backer of the military and the Second Amendment—he's a fine human being. As Altoona Police Chief six years ago, the day my wife's 19-year-old son died from complications of spinal muscle atrophy, he was the first to respond. He's worked on a much-needed expansion of mental health services in our area and has listened patiently to my concerns about Covid-19.

In his yard, no POTUS campaign signs have joined those for him and Derrick Van Orden, the Republican candidate for Congress. Recently, for understandable reasons, he erected a sign that says, "Back the Blue." Does he realize that many black people see such messages as racially coded, taking sides against Black Lives Matter, and derogating BLM?

Tuesday morning in my office, I talked politics with two POTUS supporters, both men in their 60s. The first wore his graying hair past his shoulders—late Jerry Garcia without the beard—and lives alone in the woods west of Eau Claire.

The last time I'd seen him, he faced sentencing for allegedly shooting his twelve-gage shotgun at a crop duster he'd deemed to have flown too low over his house. The pilot, who claimed my patient had put two holes in his plane, called 911, whereupon a SWAT team broke down his door and arrested him. The charges were dropped, I learned at his appointment, because there wasn't proof that my patient—who admits to brandishing his shotgun at the pilot but denies shooting at him—discharged his gun. He got off with an $800 fine for possession of a roach clip and a stash of marijuana.

I washed my hands, and he removed his shirt before I examined him, which is when I noticed a TRUMP 2020 ball cap hanging on back of the exam room door.

"What do you like about Trump?" I asked with a glance at the hat.

"He's a bully," he said. "And I think that's what we need."

I nodded, not out of agreement but to create fellow feeling, and he tried—ineffectually, in my view—to buttress his argument. Finally—he talks slowly, measuring his words, perhaps my non-verbal response to them—I said that, in my opinion, our great presidents have shown outstanding leadership in difficult times. Washington, for example. Lincoln. FDR.

His turn to nod. Before 2016, when he'd cast his vote for POTUS, my patient had twice voted for Obama. "My father"—a lifelong Democrat, he said—"would be throwing stones at me."

I suggested that COVID was a political gift to any leader with a semblance of competence and compassion, citing Angela Merkel as exemplary.

Another nod of his head.

"In my opinion," I said, "Trump is the worst president in the history of the United States."

"I'd have to agree with you," my patient said.

But he still plans to vote for him.

My next POTUS-backing patient—of which I was aware—has spent the past two decades meeting the needs of down-on-their-luck men. Trained as an engineer, he retired in his late 40s and felt God's calling to move to Eau Claire, where he purchased a dilapidated hotel. He rents its 25 units, at $15 a night, to impoverished men.

Mental health and/or substance abuse issues are nearly universal. The rooms are always full. He's reached out to other homeless men, brought them blankets, told them the Lake Street Bridge is safe to sleep under. In 2011, he helped open the Sojourner House for homeless men. Did he mind if I asked for whom he would vote?

"Trump," he said without hesitation. Neither did I have to ask him to elaborate. "We need his good business mind," he said, "and his strength on foreign policy."

He didn't ask my opinion.

After morning clinic, my wife and I drove an hour north to kayak the Flambeau River. En route, as farmland yielded to forest, we counted over 100 POTUS signs and only one family endorsing his opponent. In that yard, three Biden signs were wrapped around tree trunks, as if needing their support, as if unable to stand on their own. (Not far from the truth, maybe, with the plethora of Biden signs vanishing in the dark of the night, including that of my 90-year-old parents.)

As we paddled, though, the sun was summertime-warm, the sky and river a vivid blue. Red and yellow reflected in the glassy water, which doubled the glory of the maple trees. Sandhill cranes, in pairs or small groups, soared above. A flock of geese took flight, wings churning the water white.

Rounding a bend, in the distance downstream, appeared a pair of white dots. They floated away from us, lazy like the current. We approached, attempting stealth, but before we could draw near, they lifted off the water. The tundra swans flew toward us, one behind the other, seeming to gain speed, white plumage bracketed by black bills and feet. We watched until they were out of sight.

Four years ago, the polls were wrong. Then and now, if POTUS yard signs shooting up like spring cornstalks are indicative, momentum is shifting his way. Whether or not he wins, more than 60 million Americans will cast their votes for him. At his rallies, thousands will risk their lives to cheer his bullying and bathe in his hate-filled speech.

To a person, his supporters watch Fox; scores have told me this election cycle, and in the last, whenever I've asked. They don't read left-leaning blogs. They might not buy books or go to libraries. But most of them are inherently good.

And some are great.

Bishop Michael Curry, who presided at the wedding of Prince Harry and Meghan Markle, has a new book out entitled *Love Is The Way: Holding On To Hope In Troubling Times*. This past weekend, on NPR, he was asked how he would counsel Harry and Meghan, who've had their own challenges, were they to seek his advice.

"Keep your head up and love," he said. "Love not as a sentiment, but as a commitment. Love that seeks the good—the welfare of others, as well as the self. Unselfish, sacrificial—that is the love that can change the world."

Small comfort, you say?

Maybe not.

ONE MAN, ONE VOTE

October 18

"I don't want to die."

My 80-something patient appeared less frail than either her words or medical history would suggest. Her short and graying hair held a remembrance of a raven past. A mask concealed her mouth and nose, into which oxygen flowed, the tubing disappearing beneath the face covering.

In the hospital, where everyone is masked, one's attention is drawn to another's eyes. Hers were brown, from which frown lines radiated like spokes on a wheel. I saw fear in her eyes, but they were also resolute.

Outside the door of room 12 in our emergency department, before walking in to see her, I'd removed my yellow surgical mask, replaced it with an N95 and layered the surgical mask on top of the N95. Next I put on gloves, slipped into a gown, tying it behind my neck—challenging for a person with limited dexterity, one reason I didn't choose a career in surgery—before finally donning my transparent face shield, securing it around my noggin' like a hockey goalie's mask.

She lay on a gurney, head propped up at 45 degrees, and I pulled up a stool at her side. My new patient was my old neighbor, I discovered; she lives in an apartment complex mere blocks from my house. "Mary" tested positive for the virus one week earlier. Enrolled in Mayo's COVID home monitoring program, she was keeping an eye on her oxygen levels, which had stayed stable, thanks to O2 that flowed 24/7 into her nose, needed because of longstanding COPD.

That morning at 4, she'd awakened struggling to breathe. After dialing 911, an ambulance took her to the hospital.

A friend in the apartment building tested positive three days after Mary did. Though the two of them were careful otherwise, when they drove to get groceries together, neither wore a mask. Mary wasn't sure who'd infected whom. Perhaps one of them got the virus from another resident in their complex who'd also come down with the disease. Mary had every COVID symptom: chills, sweats, cough, head and body aches, fatigue, shortness of breath, loss of taste and smell. At the onset of her symptoms, she had diarrhea, which is also common.

Mary took me in, paused for a moment before saying, "My son had nice curly hair, just like you."

I heard "had," past tense, but didn't want to assume. "He *had* curly hair?"

"He's no longer here."

"I'm sorry. What happened?"

"He was killed in a motorcycle accident. He and his brother-in-law, my daughter's husband."

"I'm so sorry. Do you have other children?"

"I had four. There's only one left. Delores is 62. She's my rock."

I gave her time.

"My other son committed suicide, at 23. And my first child was stillborn at full term," she added, hinting at obstetrical complications, perhaps malpractice.

I waited, again. "You've had a hard life. Did you work outside of the home?"

"I stayed home when my children were young. When they went to school, I became a crossing guard. My husband died at 47. Cirrhosis of the liver. He was an alcoholic. Not a nice man." She paused for a moment. "After he died, I cleaned houses." Her words were matter-of-fact, expression emotionless. "I never married again. Once was enough for me."

"I understand."

She took a breath and asked, "What are my chances?"

Her age and emphysema put her at high risk of death. But her vital signs were stable, and her chest x-ray looked okay. Her lungs, though, when I listened with my scope, wheezed musically when she exhaled, and she gasped for breath whenever she coughed.

"You probably have a 25 percent chance of dying," I said, sensing she'd take the news with equanimity, which she did. "But that means you have a 75 percent chance of surviving," I quickly added. "And we'll do everything possible to take good care of you."

"Thank you for trying to help me," she said.

I took off and threw away my gloves, removed my gown, placed it in the hamper, washed my hands and walked out of the room. At the face-shield cleaning station, I put on a new pair of gloves—to protect my hands from bleach in the wipes—and swabbed my shield clean. Next I tossed my surgical mask before removing my N95 and, holding my breath, quickly slipped on a new surgical one. After sanitizing my hands, I was ready for the next patient.

The week before last, in morning huddle, one of my Republican colleagues said it wasn't clear what was causing Wisconsin's surge of infections.

"I don't think it's too hard to sort out," I said. "College students are back and partying; the weather's getting colder, moving everybody inside; there are Trump signs everywhere, especially in the countryside, and science deniers who won't wear masks; the Wisconsin Tavern League will keep bars open regardless, no matter the cost in human lives; and conservatives on the state Supreme Court won't let Governor Evers shut them down, something that, facing this situation, any sane society would do. Plus," I added, trying to keep my heart rate down (that all of the above is happening really bothers me) "people are sick and tired of keeping their distance and wearing masks."

From our local leadership two days ago: "The trends over the past week have been alarming both in our communities and within our hospitals. Daily we are seeing new records for Covid-19 testing, confirmed positives, percent of positive tests, and hospitalizations."

Today we have 31 COVID patients in our region's five hospitals, most of them in Eau Claire, where four are in intensive care, three of these on ventilators.

The dreaded and long-planned-for surge has come to pass; last week, I was deployed to the hospital, a gig I've volunteered to do often in the coming weeks. My new colleagues in hospital medicine, the vast majority immigrants, have been awesome: helpful, welcoming, and patient with my EHR incompetence. Together with nurses and pharmacists, often joined by social workers and therapists, I'm part of a team that coordinates each patient's care.

All patients admitted with COVID get e-consults from infectious disease doctors in Rochester, who relay treatment recommendations remotely within an hour. In the 28 years since it began, the benefits of the merger with Mayo have never been more apparent.

The virus maims and kills through a combination of three basic mechanisms: direct tissue damage, an over-robust immune response to infection, and blood clots. Each patient is treated with prophylactic blood thinners, and blood CRP and d-dimer levels—markers for systemic inflammation and clotting, respectively—are closely followed.

This past week, each of my three new COVID admissions, upon Rochester's recommendation, received the antiviral Remdesivir. (It will be interesting to see if this advice continues, considering the WHO's 11,000-patient study, published online two days ago, that concluded Remdesivir provided no clinical benefit.) None of my patients received dexamethasone—the potent anti-inflammatory steroid given to POTUS, which may have disinhibited his atrophied pre-frontal cortex yet more—because they were clinically stable and their CRPs were only modestly up. Two days ago, I discharged a lady in her late 80's to her daughter's care after she'd completed the five-day intravenous antiviral course. She did well in the hospital, and her prognosis is good.

Earlier in the week, I pulled into the parking lot of a busy intersection on the south side of Eau Claire, a hotbed of pro-POTUS activity, festooned by placards and flags. From the beds of each of two big black pickups flew a trio of Trump flags. I hopped out of my Subaru, on top of which sat my sleek and flashy pink and blue paddleboard, and approached a 60s-ish couple. The man was short, with a plus-size paunch, his bushy beard a graying red. He wore faded jeans, his black leather vest inscribed Bikers for Trump. I'd come from work, dressed in slacks and a button-down.

The man was retired. He'd run a salvage yard and an auto repair shop before switching to installing HVAC systems, mostly for clinics and hospitals, the last seventeen years of his career. He and the lady gazed up at the roof of the building next to the lot, where young men erected mammoth POTUS signs.

"I was hoping to talk with one of the men who own one of those trucks," I said with a nod at a vehicle.

"I own one," the man said.

"Great!" I said. "Can I talk with you?"

"What about?"

"What do you like about Trump?"

"My freedoms," he said. "And we gotta clean the swamp."

"Drain the swamp," echoed the woman, nodding.

"How about the virus," I said. "What are your thoughts?"

"It's a silent world war." When I gave him a quizzical look, he added, "It's been proven that the Chinese made this virus. They did it to pay back Trump for what he's done to them. And you can't trust Biden. What's he done in 47 years?"

"Do you think Biden is more liberal than other Democrats?"

"Biden's just a puppet. He's just there to have Ka-MA-la Harris take over. He'll be there three months before he turns it over to her. President Ka-MA-la and Vice President Nancy Pelosi. How you gonna live with that? Americans won't stand for socialism. I mean, we won't take it. All you need is 51 percent."

"What if it's 55-45?" I asked.

"Ain't no way. Something's crooked if that's how it comes out. Everyone I talk to is for Trump."

At this stage of our conversation, it might not have been clear to him that everyone he'd talked to didn't include me, but pointing this out seemed superfluous.

"What about masks?" I asked.

"What about them?"

"To prevent the virus from spreading." Neither he nor I had one on. But we were outside, and the wind was blowing.

He shook his head. "Ain't gonna help. You telling me someone can spread it without any symptoms?"

"Yes," I said. "And I'm a doctor."

He threw his head back and laughed. "Ain't no way! I done my research."

Something on which we both could agree: on November 3, he and I get one vote.

COVID VS. POTUS:
THE VIRUS WINS

November 2

"Don't be afraid of it," said POTUS, on his release from Walter Reed Army Hospital following three days of treatment for the virus he'd worked so hard to ignore. "You're going to beat it," he added triumphantly, as if COVID had done him no harm.

After Marine One landed on the White House lawn, POTUS lumbered up a few steps to the balcony. Visibly short of breath, he stood to his full height, adjusted his navy suit coat, and ripped off his mask, which proved tricky to put into his coat pocket, as if unwilling to be shoved offstage. The POTUS whose bone spurs had kept him out of Vietnam did his best John Wayne, an actor playing a tough guy, flicking two thumbs up for the clicking cameras, like a gunslinger drawing a pair of six shooters. The helicopter revved in the background, unseen rotors whirred, and POTUS's orange-gray pompadour fluttered like aspen leaves in a like breeze. Before walking into the presidential residence, he waved goodbye to the press, the virus, and his political career.

Three days later, the editors of the *New England Journal of Medicine*, the most prestigious medical journal in the world, said, "Covid-19 has created a crisis throughout the world. The crisis has produced a test of leadership. With no good options to combat a novel pathogen, countries were forced to make hard choices about how to respond. Here in the United States, our leaders have failed that test. They have taken a crisis and turned it into a tragedy."

Such a statement was unprecedented in the NEJM's 208-year history. "An outbreak that has disproportionately affected communities of color has exacerbated the tensions associated with inequality," the editors said, adding that "although it is impossible to project the precise number of American lives lost because of weak and inappropriate policies, it is at least in the tens of thousands in a pandemic that has already killed more Americans than any conflict since World War II. Anyone else who recklessly squandered lives… in this way would be suffering legal consequences."

The editors concluded by saying, "Truth is neither liberal nor conservative. When it comes to the response to the largest public health crisis of our time, our current political leaders have demonstrated that they are dangerously incompetent. We should not abet them and enable the deaths of thousands more Americans by allowing them to keep their jobs."

How do we know that governmental incompetence has caused the deaths of tens of thousands of Americans? Of course POTUS disagrees, saying, "I couldn't have done it any better." (Narcissists never can.) Can we know who's telling the truth? POTUS or the NEJM?

A study published in *JAMA* four days later, on Oct. 12, compared death and disease caused by COVID in the U.S. to that borne by 18 other affluent countries, grouped into low, medium, and high COVID mortality from the onset of the pandemic through Sept. 19. The Netherlands, France, Spain, Sweden, Italy, the UK, and Belgium joined the U.S. as high mortality nations, defined as > 25 COVID deaths/100,000 people. Next, the researchers looked at deaths from June 7 through Sept. 19, allowing for lag time after the implementation of initiatives to stem each country's initial viral surge.

The results were striking. Between June 7 and Sept. 19, the U.S. had more than five times the COVID mortality of six of the seven nations. (America had more than 270 % more deaths from COVID than the seventh, Sweden, whose approach to the virus, which Mark Meadows suggests we shouldn't even try to contain, has been similarly laissez faire.)

In other words, perhaps POTUS can be forgiven for not learning a lesson from the Chinese in January, the Italians in February, or Governor Cuomo in March, but by April any leader worth his spray tan should have realized COVID was nothing to sneeze at.

In another study published that same day in *JAMA*, researchers calculated excess American deaths between March 1 and August 1. Though death rates from year to year are remarkably consistent, there were 20 percent more deaths than anticipated—225,530 of them to be exact—and only 2/3 of these (a total of 150,541 deaths) were definitively attributed to COVID. Researchers postulate that the 75,000 unaccounted-for deaths were either secondary to unrecognized COVID infections or caused by health care disruptions the virus precipitated, including people choosing not to seek care for serious issues such as stroke and heart attack.

After POTUS announced his COVID diagnosis, Merriam-Webster reported a 30,000 percent increase in searches for *schadenfreude*.

Kansas Gov. Laura Kelly, a Democrat, enacted a state-wide mask mandate in July. Counties could opt out, and 82 of 105 did. Since then, the incidence of COVID in counties with mask mandates was half of that in counties without. (GPS data from cellphones showed no difference in mobility between residents of counties with and without mask mandates.)

Last week, a patient told me he was wearing a mask as he drove from his home, window down, to run an errand. Pulling up to a stop sign, a man working in his yard at the intersection yelled, "You people and your fucking masks!" before flipping him off.

The University of Washington estimates that 95 percent compliance with a nationwide indoor mask mandate could save 100,000 American lives by the end of February.

Last week, I drove with a friend to fish steelhead in Michigan. En route, driving through Chicago, we listened to Illinois Gov. J.B. Pritzker's COVID update, broadcast daily at 2:30 p.m. on WBEZ.

To fight the virus, Illinois has been divided into 11 regions. If any region shows an increase in COVID activity coupled with a simultaneous decease in hospital capacity, or if the seven-day average of positive tests exceeds 8 percent on three successive days, mitigation strategies are implemented and enforced by the state police. If Tier 1 tactics don't work, the state ratchets up to Tier 2, which, among other restrictions, bans indoor dining or bar service. Illinois has extended a $220 million aid package to affected businesses.

In Wisconsin currently, the seven-day average of positive tests is 29.5 percent.

POTUS signs and flags littered the banks of the Muskegon River like the sycamore leaves that floated lazily along its surface, clinging to our hooks, clogging the jet engine of our boat. In the river town of Newaygo, costumed parents and kids, POTUS signs in yards, sallied forth to trick or treat. The "Trump Unity Truck," *YMCA* blaring on loud speakers, cruised the main drag, honking support for the 45th President. On the drive back to Wisconsin, on a blustery Sunday, POTUS stalwarts flew flags on an overpass above I-94.

Nate Silver says that if POTUS carries Pennsylvania, where polls suggest he's down a mere 5 percent, he could win.

Along with the Dakotas, Wisconsin is conducting an experiment: As the weather cools, how much death and suffering will COVID inflict without a scrap of state-sanctioned mitigation? Conservatives on the Wisconsin Supreme Court? What do you think?

This week I'm back in the hospital, where I rounded on a patient in the ICU, a man in his late 40s. Yesterday, he'd been shopping in the Twin Cities with his wife when he developed severe chest pain that moved up to his jaw and down his arms. He'd been diagnosed with COVID 10 days earlier, shortness of breath from that infection was suddenly worse, and he broke out in a sweat.

The man presented to a rural Wisconsin hospital, where blood tests confirmed myocardial injury: a heart attack. After being airlifted to our Eau Claire hospital, an angiogram revealed normal coronary arteries. The virus caused his chest pain and heart injury, though the mechanism isn't clear.

The patient I'd written about Oct. 18, the elderly lady who didn't want to die, fared well at first. But on her third afternoon in the hospital, she went downhill. She decided against life support, and early the next morning my patient died.

On Oct. 6, the day after leaving the hospital, POTUS announced he wouldn't pursue fiscal stimulus but would focus instead on the Supreme Court confirmation of Amy Coney Barrett. Why he couldn't walk and chew gum simultaneously was left unexplained.

Two days later, talking with Fox News' Maria Bartiromo the morning after the vice-presidential debate, POTUS called Kamala Harris a "monster" and said his Vice had "destroyed her." That same day, though trailing in the polls, POTUS announced he wouldn't debate Joe Biden one week hence. During this time, he was being treated with dexamethasone, which is known to impair judgement.

"Don't be afraid of it," said POTUS of the virus that, as of today, has killed more than 231,000 Americans. "You're going to beat it."

History will show that COVID beat *him*. Tomorrow, the votes will be tallied. On the results, we will breathlessly wait.

THE ROAD BACK
TO HEALTH

November 15

"I don't want to go to Rochester," my patient said, his voice muffled. "This is the best I've felt in days."

Late morning, in the emergency department's room 10, I sat on a stool at his side. "Danny" lay on a gurney, his head propped up at 45 degrees. In his early 60s, a year older than me, he tops the scales at over 300 pounds. His uncombed black hair is flecked with silver (perhaps like me, he's late for a haircut), a modest beard more gray. With each breath he initiated, a BiPap mask cinched tight over nose and mouth forced oxygen into his lungs.

But his appearance backed up his words. He looked comfortable, not laboring to breathe. Besides mask and setting, we could have been sitting at a local restaurant sipping the coffee that he ground for a living.

Usually the eyes of a critically ill patient evince fear or fatigue. But Danny's brown orbs seemed content, with a hint of a mischievous glint. Isn't it silly, they seemed to suggest, for us to be meeting under these strange circumstances?

When I told him he'd likely end up on a ventilator, perhaps before the end of the day, his eyes grew moist.

"I don't understand," he said.

"You're on 100 percent oxygen," I said, "And that machine is helping you breathe. If it's not enough, we'll have to put you on a ventilator."

"You mean with a tube jammed down my throat?"

I nodded. "If it becomes necessary, do you want us to do it?"

He hesitated. "I dunno."

Further discussion clarified that he was more uncertain about needing a ventilator than about using one, should the need arise. I pushed hard for him to agree to life support. Without a ventilator, he'd likely die. With its help, he'd have a decent chance to pull through.

"Okay," he said.

Two and a half weeks earlier, per protocol before a lymph node biopsy, he'd tested COVID negative. Not long after the biopsy, he started to cough. For a day or two, he lost his sense of taste and smell. Though his breathing was off a little, he wasn't alarmed.

Danny denied chest pain, didn't have head or body aches. He had a low-grade fever of which he'd not been aware. His only complaints, really, were weakness and fatigue. He was usually healthy, he said, with plenty of energy. To feel exhausted was odd.

One of the many tragedies of our COVID surge—of COVID surges everywhere—is that family members aren't permitted in the hospital, a policy implemented to protect patients and staff. I doffed my PPE, walked out of room 10, and called his wife.

"I couldn't get him to go to the hospital," she said. "For the last three days, all he did was sleep in his chair. And he was getting confused, not making sense."

Danny's oxygen levels were dangerously low, low enough, in other diseases, to almost always cause extreme air hunger, low enough to scramble his brain. Often in COVID pneumonia, however, for unclear reasons, the respiratory rate fails to ramp up. It's as if the virus affects the brainstem, which tells the lungs not to breathe, and the cerebral cortex doesn't recognize the condition's severity, even to the point of death. There's a name for patients like Danny: happy hypoxics.

His chest CT scan showed extensive ground-glass opacities in both lungs, COVID's radiographic hallmark, but not until the next day did results of a nasal swab, taken within minutes of him being wheeled into room 10, confirm the diagnosis.

Several hours later, Danny's condition hadn't changed. He needed an ICU bed, but none was available. (This past week, we've been on full hospital bypass most mornings, into mid-afternoon, when some patients are discharged, freeing up beds. By car or ambulance, patients keep coming to the emergency department, where they sit for hours before a bed opens up.) A pulmonologist who'd consulted virtually wanted the patient transferred to Rochester, explaining that Danny risked crashing and burning in the middle of the night. In that event, to emergently intubate his trachea, and flip his obese body prone, would not only be difficult but potentially life-threatening. If bad led to worse, better for him to be where such high-level procedures were more routinely performed.

But the ER doctor, a remarkable mother of three with board certifications both in critical care and emergency medicine, thought he'd be safe in a non-ICU bed. I went back to room 10 to break the proverbial tie, which is when Danny nixed the transfer to Rochester.

The discussion became moot, because later that afternoon an ICU bed opened up. The next morning Danny went downhill and was put on a ventilator. When he lay supine, not even 100 percent oxygen pumped into his lungs was enough. Flipped on his stomach, though, he received just enough oxygen to keep him alive.

After working these past two weeks in the hospital, I have the weekend off. When I drove to my office to tie up loose ends, an NBC crew from New York City was interviewing Mayo leadership in the parking lot.

Small wonder. COVID cases in Wisconsin have set records each of the last three days. Despite being one-third as populous, the Badger State is seeing more cases a day than NYC at the peak of its surge. Hospitals are close to their breaking points; starting yesterday, patients may not receive needed care. For the next month and beyond, it's projected that an already grim situation will only get worse: More hospitalizations, more patients on ventilators, 3,500 additional Wisconsinites dead of COVID by the end of the year. In addition, because of the squeeze on hospitals, more patients will die of non-COVID causes than would have otherwise.

In the U.S., population 331 million, new cases Nov. 13 set a record at 184,000, with 1,389 added deaths. The same statistics from other countries: Germany, pop. 83 million: 15,920 new cases and 115 new deaths; Canada, pop. 37 million: 3,585 cases and 60 deaths; South Korea, pop. 52 million: 205 and four; China, pop. 1.3 billion: 18 and zero; Australia, pop. 25 million: eight and zilch. Because we did so poorly controlling COVID this summer, more virus was circulating at the beginning of fall, and off to the races it went.

China waged ruthless war on the virus in January, Italy locked down in February, and New York City took a number of tacks in March. Now in Wisconsin, we're conducting an experiment: As winter approaches, how many people will die of the virus in the total absence of government-sanctioned mitigation? No enforcement of mask mandates, no restrictions on bars, no limitations on schools or mobility. It's reminiscent of the Tuskegee syphilis study, where white researchers, at a time when syphilis could be cured, "studied" its natural history in black men, which often progressed to dementia or death.

A recent study of 5,000 Houston patients confirmed that COVID is mutating. During the spring surge, 71 percent of patients infected with COVID had a mutation called D614G in the spike protein, which allows the virus to wedge its way into a cell. By the time of the second, summertime surge, 99.9 percent of viral genomes contained the mutation. The most likely explanation: D614G facilitates cellular entry, making COVID more contagious.

Joe Biden is president-elect. By the time all of the ballots are counted, he will have won by roughly six million votes. The 306-232 Electoral College tally is precisely the same as four years ago, when POTUS, despite losing the popular vote by 2.8 million, proclaimed a "landslide" victory.

In 2016 POTUS became president because of a cumulative margin of 77,000 votes in three states: Michigan, Pennsylvania, and Wisconsin. In 2020 the collective gap was almost the same in four: Georgia, Nevada, Arizona, and Wisconsin. If Stacey Abrams hadn't registered swarms of democrats; if Harry Reid's political machine hadn't turned out Las Vegas culinary workers; if POTUS hadn't gotten into a pissing match with Cindy McCain; and if Wisconsin hadn't hearkened back to its progressive roots, POTUS would have won a second term. In these four states, if one in 300 Biden voters instead had marked their ballot for Trump, the outcome would have been reversed.

Seventy-nine percent of POTUS voters cast their ballot for him, rather than against Biden, while the priority for 51 percent of Biden supporters was to oust the sitting president. During the campaign, the profusion of POTUS signs and flags throughout the rural heartland advertised a deep and abiding love for an inept sociopath. Yesterday, thousands of his supporters marched in Washington, arguing that the election had been stolen. If POTUS says something, however demonstrably false, Americans by the tens of millions believe him.

More than 73 million of our fellow citizens voted for someone who is manifestly unfit for the office of president, a man who refuses to separate lies from the truth, a self-serving huckster whose arrogance and incompetence has led to the loss of tens of thousands of American lives.

Democracy is precarious. Facts rest on a shaky foundation.

For three days in the ICU, Danny's survival was no less insecure. Every time he lay on his back, his oxygen levels plummeted. But when the nurses flipped him face down, his condition stabilized. The next five days, though, he could tolerate lying supine, and his respiratory therapist started weaning him off the ventilator. Early this morning, the tube was taken out of his trachea, and Danny is breathing on his own.

Now, like the nation in which he resides, he can take the first steps, begin the long journey, on the road back to health.

NOTES AND ACKNOWLEDGMENTS:

To preserve patient privacy, throughout the book, names and identifying information have been changed.

I'm proud of my son Erik, whose artistry graces the cover. Jan Wisner did expert copy editing. Don Wisner urged me to turn my blog into a book. Many readers of my blog offered encouragement. I'm especially grateful for kind words from friends and colleagues at the Mayo Clinic, both in Eau Claire and in Rochester, and at UW-Eau Claire. Special shout outs to Jan Larsen, and Drs. Bill Rupp, Chris Roberts, Charles Rohren, Sandeep Basu, and Paul Thomas.

Monica was the book's biggest fan. Though we're no longer together, words can't express my appreciation for her patience, love, and support.